What Patie
about Dr. Bonnie

Marie, thank you for your trust with your health. Bonnie

Before I had high blood pressure, low energy, heartburn, and many other health issues. I was a very unhealthy eater and obese. I used to get sick every time someone else got sick with the flu or a cold. My daughter was born premature. She had bad eczema. She also has gastrointestinal issues as well as sinus issues.

Now I feel fantastic. My energy level is high. My blood pressure has stabilized. I'm losing weight. Health improvement has encouraged me and made it easier for me to eat healthy. I no longer get sick. Last year there were multiple family members who all got the flu or a cold and it did not touch me. Health improvement has definitely changed my life. My daughter's eczema has improved, her sinuses have improved, and she no longer has gastrointestinal issues. I wish I would have started sooner.

Robin Nolan

I was struggling with low energy, fatigue, dizziness, and eczema. It was so severe I was not able to keep up with my work. I also had chronic UTIs that the specialist (Western medicine) was not able to stop.

All my symptoms are gone, and I feel better than I ever have. I have tons of energy; my eczema is gone. Best of all my UTIs are gone, and I am able to work longer and harder than when I was in my twenties. We also had been trying for years to have a baby. Once I was healthy, we were pregnant in three months. My dreams came true at last! Thank you, Dr. Bonnie.

Katie Garrett, horse trainer

I was diagnosed with interstitial cystitis in 2011 and had resolved it for five years. I came to Dr. Bonnie to deal with IC symptoms, detox, and hormonal changes due to perimenopause. I had many food sensitivities, digestion problems, sleep issues. I found out that I needed to change my diet more specifically and work on clearing toxins like mold, yeast, environmental issues, etc.

I've resolved many issues like clearing out underlying toxicity. Through muscle testing I can determine what and how much supplementation to do. Dr. Bonnie is very sensitive and tuned in. She is able to find subtleties other doctors could not find. I have learned to be more connected to what my body needs and to trust it because of the work I've done with Dr. Bonnie.

Belen Avellan

I was hospitalized two to three times a year with severe abdominal pain and bloating. I was taking antidepressants for three to four years. In the few years prior to starting I gained twenty-five pounds and had hot flashes thanks to menopause. Regularly I experienced back and hip pain. Once to twice a year prior to starting I developed bronchitis.

I have not been hospitalized for three years. No further episodes of bronchitis and have stopped my allergy medication. After seeing Dr. Bonnie for a year, I was able to gradually wean off my antidepressants. If I experience joint pain, it is seldom related to the activities I perform. I am more aware of my body and its responses to foods.

Jennifer Aspen, occupational therapist

I was on Nexium for acid reflux, and XYTec (a twenty-four-hour antihistamine) for seasonal allergies. It made me less sharp. Was eating too much sugar but wasn't fat.

I'm down fifteen pounds, taking no drugs of any kind. No seasonal allergies, no acid reflux. Feel sharp and energetic.

Peter Gregory, retired entrepreneur

When I first started my wellness journey with Dr. Bonnie, I was in bed four days a week and considering fighting for disability. I felt hopeless and physically done with life in general. Sleeping was the only thing I actually enjoyed. Everything I ate I reacted to. My stomach was hard and constantly bloated. I felt isolated and alone.

Dr. Bonnie is my angel. She gave me hope and sincerely cared about my wellness success. Her eyes showed caring, sympathy, and love. I've never had a doctor make me feel this way. Dr. Juul has held my hand as I took baby steps through my healing journey. A year later we are still walking together. I feel so much better, never take naps, and eat close to normal again. Dr. Juul will work hard for you.

Sherrie Malone, business educator

Escape the Medical
Merry-Go-Round, Reclaim
Your Health, and Live a
Long and Healthy Life

VIM
AND
VIGOR

DR. BONNIE JUUL

ISBN paperback: 978-1-958181-01-0
ISBN hardcover: 978-1-958181-02-7
ISBN ebook: 978-1-958181-03-4
ISBN audiobook: 978-1-958181-04-1

Published by Dortheus Publishing, www.dortheuspublishing.com, Carbondale, IL.

Contact the author at DortheusPublishing@gmail.com.

Contents

Part II

The 3 Contributors to Health That You Can Control

Part II

Working with a Professional

Introduction

"If you haven't got your health, you haven't got anything."
Count Rugen, *The Princess Bride*

This book is specifically for you if you want answers for your health outside of the answers you are getting in the medical system.

If you are like most people entering this journey, at least one of three concerns has brought you here:

1. You are desperate to get answers where the medical system didn't give them to you,

2. You have a spiritual belief and understanding that we are meant to be healthy, or

3. You have come to realize that the people in our world aren't getting any healthier—even though you see them

spending a significant amount of time, money, and effort on their health and healthcare. Autoimmune disease, heart disease, new diseases, diseases that were once affecting a few are now affecting the many and being normalized.

Maybe you don't want to support the pharmaceutical companies, maybe you just don't want to be sick. Maybe you don't want to be the person who slowly declines before they finally die.

Maybe your child has a medical injury and you can't get help. Maybe you're just scared for the health of your children because you want to see them spend more time playing and less time suffering or in the doctor's office.

The majority of people in the world expect to have their bodies age in such a way that they will spend most of their time navigating doctor visits, needing more and more medications, having more and more procedures, and ultimately experiencing gradually declining health with little to no independence for the last few years of life.

This isn't for you.

There is, obviously, a certain level of security for those believing what they are told. And misery loves company, so a lot of people get together and share about their medications and suffering.

If you're willing to give up that way of bonding with others, then this approach to health and lifestyle could be for you.

Just a warning: You have to be made of something a little stronger and a little different from the average person to follow this plan. You'll be just outside the norms of society. People don't get this. They also don't understand just how great you can feel and how it is to focus on living life and enjoying life instead of suffering.

Imagine that. No suffering!

Fortunately, you are joining a growing group of people living extraordinarily healthy lives.

Welcome. And congratulations on looking and living outside the box.

The Scope of This Book

This book is based on my many years of experience helping thousands of people restore their health. After decades of trying all the fads, doing the trial and error of recommendations myself, in the following pages I share the patterns of what all successful programs have in common. It's what works.

There is also a certain way that the people who get better interact with the material they are learning so that they get the results they are looking for.

Let's look at the three basic types of interactions people have with this type of information, and then we'll get into the meat of it.

Readers will interact with this information in a variety of ways. However, there are loosely three categories of interaction. Depending on where you fit most closely, you can see where your results might be.

This information is at the beginning of the book because, depending on where you fall, this book might not be the greatest benefit to you, so it wouldn't be worth your time to work through it.

The Get-It-Done Person: This person is determined to improve and then maintain their health level and independence over the years. She is willing to do what she needs to fight the aging process. She wants to know what she needs to do to get stronger and healthier, and she just does it. She seems to defy the odds and is perhaps a bit of a mystery to those around her, often considered lucky by those not realizing the conscientiousness and work put into maintaining such health. She is going to acknowledge the information that she already knows and look for the information she doesn't so that she can implement it, communicate if something doesn't quite work right, and ask the question, "How can I take the information given to me and use it so I can get the result I want?" This person has excellent results.

The It's-Good-Enough Person: She dabbles a little bit with ideas here and there, takes some recommendations, but not a lot, has to reduce activities and limits what she can do, plays around with different diets, is still active, may or may not be taking pain pills regularly, and has the typical decline of health expected for people as they age, but is likely doing a little bit better than some of her peers. This person expects that suffering is a part of getting older but will do a little bit here and there to try and get better. This person has moderate results, will probably be on one or two medications, and is happy with this. This person will have moderate results.

The I'm-Too-Busy Person: *Someone just tell me what to do, and I'll consider it if I don't have to make changes.* This person does what she is told, often when convenient or if it doesn't interfere with her life.

She is unwilling to make any dietary or lifestyle changes. She rarely or loosely investigates solutions, focusing mainly on the problem and the pain. When considering solutions, she looks to see how convenient it is to her. Whether or not she wants to be on medications, she will likely end up on some at some point. She may bounce from possible solution to possible solution, rarely committing 100 percent to anything. She prefers to have someone tell her what to do and then not have to think about it. This person is best served staying with the medical route, and this book may be a waste of her time.

Obviously, the results will be different for each person as these are sweeping generalizations. Most of us are somewhere along a gradient. And none of these is the right way or wrong way to do it. Each of these dietary and lifestyle changes is perfect for the person doing them. The people who will benefit most from what I am writing in this book are in the first two groups.

The more you are willing to do for yourself, the better your results.

As more people use this information and it becomes normalized, it will help the health of not only you and your family but of future generations. If you are going to argue about what is in here because of the more mainstream data you have been following, then this is not for you.

On the flip side, utilizing this information puts you outside the realm of the ordinary and puts you solidly into the world of the extraordinary. Extraordinary.

If you see something or find something that you want to delve more into, the internet resources and suggested books listed at the end of this book are excellent resources. If you would like a Part 2 with more detailed information on something, please let me know at info@DrBonnieJuul.com.

Warning

If you are on medications, it may be dangerous and, yes, fatal to remove yourself from medications without a proper weaning process or before making sure that your blood tests or other tests come back normal. Be sure to check in with your healthcare practitioner if you want to integrate any of these recommendations. Always get the approval of your prescribing doctor before getting off medications. I cannot stress this enough.

If your health has declined to the degree that you need medications to stay healthy, the strategy is always to get on the medication. Then when the appropriate changes have been made, you will no longer need the medication. Pride of "not needing medications" has no place here. Your prescribing doctor can help you safely wean off your medications, if appropriate.

The recommendations in this book have worked for everyone who has used this information as a baseline and, following the recommendations, tweaked them for their unique situation. You can do the same. Since every person who has implemented these recommendations has had improvement, why not you?

Who I Am

Why should you listen to me?

I'm going to give you my background as it relates to being healthy. As far as the changes that I made, I'll share those with you as we go through the rest of the book.

At the time that I'm writing this, I have just turned fifty-three. I'm much healthier and more vital than I was twenty years ago. I exercise five or six days a week (the hard stuff: jumping around, running, lifting weights), eat well, and I'm doing awesome, actually.

And it wasn't an easy journey to get here. It was so hard that I wouldn't wish this path on my worst enemy.

I hope that this book and my story will prevent you from traveling down the path of hell that I went through. And if you're sitting in the muck of it like I was, my greatest desire is that this book gives you hope and shines a light on your pathway out.

I'm on the other side and am forever grateful. On this side of the health spectrum, you guard your health like a mama bear guards her cubs. I'm just a regular person. So, if I can do it, you can.

And here is . . .

How My Journey Started

It was 1999. I was twenty-nine years old and in a master's program for teaching English. I planned to travel the world. Teaching English would be my ticket to getting employment in whatever country I wanted to go to.

I thought about health as being slender and fit. And it was relatively easy for me. While in school, I gained a little weight, so I started eating frozen vegetables and frozen fish. I'd just put them in the microwave to heat them. I cut back on the sugar a little and increased the exercise. I drank wine with dinner, but that was my little treat. And sometimes I'd have ice cream at night. But I made sure my calories were low. And I'd lose weight.

I looked good.

For the pain I was in from previous injuries (skiing accident, flipping over on my bicycle and landing on my face, I was a leap-and-then-look kind of kid), I would just take my painkillers. Because that's what you did.

And when I had my debilitating cramps from my period every other month, I'd suffer, take the Aleve, and it usually worked. If it didn't work, I'd just suffer through.

When I say debilitating cramps, the cramps were so bad that I'd take one to two days off every other month, lying on the cool bathroom floor, crying, vomiting, having diarrhea, sweating, trying to breathe, and just waiting for the pain to get over.

If I knew then what I know now, I'd never go through that.

But mine was a normal life—my pain and suffering were part of the normal scheme of things. Everyone seemed to have something. Pills would help, and if they didn't, you were out of luck.

I was planning a regular, American life with the future of adventure thrown in.

My first job when I graduated with my master's degree in English was in South Korea. I had to take a handful of vaccines to go there. I remember when the nurse gave them to me. She showed me sheets of paper with information on them, written in fine print and using big words I didn't understand.

I didn't read it because I trusted her. She was a nurse and obviously knew more than I did. She gave me all my shots, and I didn't think anything else about it.

Fast-forward a few months to living in South Korea. Exercise was a little more uncomfortable for me. I started having trouble breathing. But I attributed it to the stress of living in another country, quite different from anywhere else I had lived.

I mostly ignored the increased discomfort because I was focused on working and experiencing life in my new home. I still mostly ate what I wanted and kept it as healthy as I understood at the time.

I was starting to have a sensitivity to certain foods. But that was something people had. So I didn't think much about it. I just tried to eat around it. If I did eat something that bothered me, I would have trouble breathing. It was annoying but manageable. I was taking it all in stride.

During my last month there, I traveled to visit a friend on a remote island in the Philippines and had to take an antimalarial drug. I took the pills for two weeks before I went, the two weeks I was there, and two weeks after.

While I was there, my body started losing control. Out of nowhere, I felt a crushing pressure come down on my chest and felt like I couldn't breathe. I thought I was going to die. I didn't want to bother my friend, so I got up in the middle of the night and put my face in the freezer so I could get a breath. It was a hot and humid place with no air conditioning. The freezer worked.

The next morning, my friend told me that a lot of people seemed to have weird reactions to the antimalarial drug, and some people just stopped taking it. One guy who was one of those super manly types got emotional and weepy on it. He had stopped taking it.

I didn't know at the time that sticking my head in the freezer was an action that I would repeat many times over the next few years. My idea at the time was what I was trained to think. It would leave my system over time. (Boy, was I wrong.)

The last time I had to stick my head in a freezer was three years ago. So twenty years after the first occurrence, it has taken me that long to figure all this out.

I moved back to the US and didn't think about my woes anymore. I got a job at a university teaching. My trouble breathing was getting worse. I was thirty years old.

I had to go up a flight of stairs to get to my office. One day I had to sit down on the steps because I couldn't make it up. A colleague asked if I was okay. I said I didn't know. So I made an appointment to get my heart checked. I went to a hospital for a stress test and whatever other tests they did. And they told me there was nothing wrong with me.

I knew there was something wrong, but I trusted them. I trusted them more than that part of me saying something was wrong. I pushed the feeling away. They knew more than I did and were medically trained. I moved on expecting that it would pass.

9/11 happened, and I decided to move near my sister in Albuquerque, NM. By now, I was starting to experience more pain. I was taking pain pills every day to manage it. I was exercising and doing yoga.

I was still convinced that exercise and some medically recommended changes in my diet were all I needed to get healthy.

By the time I got to New Mexico, the pain was severe enough that when I exercised one day, I'd have to wait three days to exercise again. The pain was too much otherwise. The pain pills weren't touching the pain at that point.

Like the story of the boiling frog in water, I barely noticed it was getting worse until I reflected on it years later.

Frog in Water: A Lesson of Remaining Unaware

The frog in boiling water story goes something like this: If you try to put a frog in boiling water, it will jump out. But if you put a frog in comfortable water and slowly increase the temperature, it won't notice. The water will eventually boil and kill the frog. He just won't notice that he's dying. I don't know if this is true, but the point gets across.

I continued to think that as long as I kept my weight down and exercised—and ate some healthy foods—I would be able to be healthy and get my health back.

My cramps were still bad and getting worse. The symptoms were the same, but now painkillers didn't help. When I went to the doctor, I was told I was infertile.

I was also starting to have significant pain in my joints. I was in so much pain that I would cry at night. I had four to five different places I would try to sleep. If I got three hours, I was lucky. I often asked God why this was happening to me and would beg to please, please, please help me.

I'd drink coffee in the morning to get me going and wine at night to calm me down. I decided to eat mainly vegetarian food in case that would help. I would eat packaged foods that said they were healthy on the label or were commonly thought of as healthy. Beans and rice, for example.

It was hell on earth, and I wasn't even thirty-five yet. But I looked really good because I exercised and ate in a way that I was told was correct. I was slender. I was fit. I looked healthy.

But I had experiences that, when I look back now, were tip-offs that something was going wrong with my health. For example, if I went to a salad bar, I'd get diarrhea within ten minutes of eating. I stopped going to them because I found out that the lettuce is sprayed with a chemical to keep it fresh looking.

That was new information for me. I started investigating.

I didn't make the connection with my diet, and no medical person ever talked to me about it. Ever. Not once.

I went to the doctor and got a blood test for sensitivities. There were only minor ones, and I was low in iodine. My doctors weren't concerned.

I didn't learn until many years later how alarming that was regarding my health and how it was linked to my pain. When the pain got bad enough, I went to a pain specialist. He took an MRI. The report came in. He told me there was nothing wrong.

I said, "Yes, there is. There is something wrong with me. I have a scar on my right butt cheek from a fall many years ago." I told him, "I have this scar here. You didn't even check that."

He said, "I'm a doctor. I have had many years of training, and there is nothing wrong with you."

"I have had my body for my entire life," I said, "and I'm telling you there is something wrong with me."

"There is nothing wrong with you. I am referring you to a psychiatrist."

He walked me over to a model of a spine and started talking about it. I didn't hear a word he said. I was completely livid.

How am I going to live like this for the rest of my life? That was it. I realized I was going to have to figure this out on my own.

I Can't Do This Anymore!

I did take what he said to heart—that the pain was in my head. But I was done with trying to take different drugs. I wanted to know why I had this pain and suffering and fix that. If I could fix that, I'd be better.

God, take me home or help me figure this out. Please. I can't do this anymore.

I leaned on Jesus because he is the greatest healer, and I had to lean on someone because I had no one in my world to lean on. No one I knew could hear what I was saying about how horrible I felt. And they either didn't believe me or just plain couldn't understand the level of suffering I was in.

Because I looked healthy.

I was so alone and lost that if suicide had been on the table for me, I probably would have done it. I had to find answers. I would end up spending thousands upon thousands of dollars and hundreds of hours getting therapies and treatments, getting trained in some, and experiencing others.

I learned that just about everything I was raised to believe would make me healthy was either making me sick or limiting how healthy I could get. It took me ten years to get healthier than people my same age, and it took ten more years to fully heal and maximize my health.

My goal and my mind were on finding the solutions. It was in 2020 when I finally, finally, knew that it was over.

Suffering. Ended.

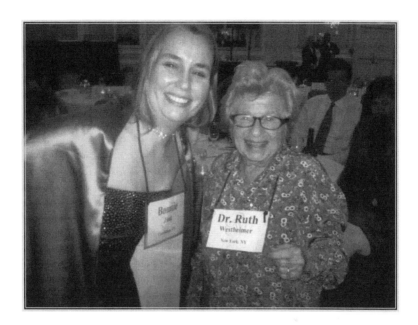

Dr. Bonnie Juul (left) with Dr. Ruth, attending the Renaissance Weekend in Charleston, South Carolina, New Year's Eve 2009. According to Dr. Bonnie, "When this picture was taken, I was in chronic pain and barely sleeping. You can see the inflammation around my face. I was living in Dallas but had traveled to New Hampshire (on my way to Charleston) for my first visit with Dr. D'Adamo, Sr., founder of the Blood Type Diet. He taught me about the common misunderstandings of food quality and how that affects health."

Why I Am Writing This Book

I'm writing this book because I know that if I can help even a few people get their health back, they will start getting themselves on track. As they need help, some will reach out to me as a resource to help them on their journey. Whether they reach out to me or not, at the very least they will be able to have a foundation of health for themselves.

When you don't feel good, it's really hard to be patient, kind, and understanding of others. Not only do you suffer, but so do your relationships.

The healthier you are, the more you can focus—without the distraction of pain and discomfort—on the things that are important to you: God, family, and friends and enjoying this beautiful world we live in.

Part I

What the Healthiest People Know about How Health Works

1

What They Never Tell You about Being Healthy

Forget everything you've heard about health and being healthy. There is an unspoken understanding of being healthy that limits what people believe is possible and, frankly, is just plain wrong.

Today's belief in what defines *healthy* keeps you tied to both the pharmaceutical industry and the need for what they are peddling. Pain, suffering, getting on more medications, trying different medications, jumping from diet to diet, surgeries, fixing failed surgeries, stress and more stress, fear, anxiety, trying to do everything—it's giving the illusion that if you do more, you'll get better.

But are you? Are you healthier today than you were last year? Or do you just have fewer symptoms because your medication is working?

The truth is, people aren't getting healthier. Quite the opposite. They are masking symptoms with medications while the disease processes are still running unchecked behind the scenes.

You have likely observed someone you care about taking medical advice and still getting sicker and sicker. Maybe it's even you.

We are on a downward spiral, and it's ultimately up to you and me to help us get out of it. The basics of what it takes to be genuinely healthy are more straightforward than you might expect. So let's get on the same page about the definition of health. And we'll work from that.

What Is Health . . . Really?

That's the question. What is the mainstream definition of health, and what does it mean? Is health working for us? Or does health need to be redefined?

The agreed-upon definition of health is essential to look at because the definition is what we all operate from. The World Health Organization website states: "Health is a state of complete physical, mental and social well-being and not merely the absence of disease or infirmity."

At first glance, it looks like something we would all want, doesn't it? But by picking the definition apart, you can see that operating from this explanation has limitations that have resulted in the continual decline of health.

"Complete physical, mental and social well-being" is a matter of perception. People define themselves as being healthy if they don't have symptoms or if medications handle the symptoms.

One of the questions on our clinic's intake form is, "On a scale of 1 to 10, how healthy are you?" If patients don't have symptoms, they rate themselves as healthy—an 8, 9, or 10. However, if you are on any medication, this means that you have one or more organs that are not functioning right. So your experience is being healthy, but in the background—behind the scenes—is a problem.

Said another way, people can have the experience of "complete physical, mental and social well-being" by having medications cover up their symptoms.

By medical standards, "the absence of disease" means that your blood tests and other medical tests are within normal limits.

Plenty of people feel terrible but also have "the absence of disease," which is why they are not getting help. The medical community can't help if they don't have a diagnosis to work from.

Here's an example: You may have gotten a blood test that indicates your health is getting worse, but the doctor says, "We'll check you in six months to see if it's worse." Usually, if you ask your doctor for recommendations on how to prevent whatever is causing the condition from getting worse, they don't have solid recommendations for you. (If you haven't had this experience, then hold on tight to your doctor, you've got a rare one.)

Infirmity means "being weak or frail." Many medications and medical devices, such as hearing aids, oxygen tanks and back braces, help people lead active lives so that their weakness and frailty don't need to be addressed through diet and exercise. Of course, medical devices are helpful, especially as health declines. But they aren't keeping people healthy and are keeping people more dependent on them.

You and I both know that we are seeing more and more lifestyle diseases, including heart disease, kidney disease, cancer, and obesity (the strongest predictor for getting COVID-19 at the time of this writing). The list goes on.

Being on medications has become the norm rather than the exception. Having an "absence of disease" is a perception that can be and is manipulated with medications and medical devices. The medications and devices fool you into thinking that you are doing better. You are told that you are doing better because your blood test (or any other test) came back better.

The tests used for medical diagnosis do not measure the presence of health but, instead, measure the absence or presence of disease. The absence of disease does not indicate your level of health. It just means you haven't gotten bad enough, or bad enough in the right way, to have a disease label and to get a medication.

Over time, these tests can show that you are heading toward disease. But they don't always.

In Real Life: The Medical Paradigm of Health

Let's look at an example of acid reflux. You have burning and belching after you eat or throughout the day. You're not sure why. You've been given some recommendations to follow for your diet, but nothing has helped.

You get on the prescribed medication, and you stop having symptoms. So you go about your business and keep living like you were living.

You take the medication for a few months, knowing that you're only supposed to use it for a short period. But every time you try to stop taking it, your symptoms come back.

Before you know it, ten years have gone by. Looks like you'll be on that drug forever.

Suppose medicine had the answers to how to reverse diseases. Would there be this many people on so many medications in a world where being sick and medicated is considered normal?

We are all conditioned to a certain type of aging in which you get worse as you get older. You get on one medication, then that has side effects, so you get on another.

The thing is: what you got on the medication for in the first place is being managed by the drug but is still getting worse in the background, so you'll need to increase that medication or get on another one at some point—or surgery.

And so on.

Fortunately, there are thousands of people aging differently. You don't hear about them because the world they live in is so far outside of the medical paradigm that many people can't even comprehend that it is possible.

We'll get into the tools that you need to get there. But before we do, let's dig into a different definition of health. One that empowers you to take charge of your health and will lead to your having health and longevity for the remainder of your life.

Other people are experiencing health and vitality throughout their daily lives and then right up until the end. So why not you?

In Real Life: The New Paradigm of Health

Let's go back to the acid reflux example, but this time in the new paradigm of health.

You figure out what foods irritate your stomach (either through trial and error, research, or muscle testing. Some basic information about muscle testing can be found at www.muscletestingbasics.com). You figure out alternatives for the foods you love and use these to give your stomach a break from the foods for at least three months.

During this time, you take supplements specifically designed to repair and restore the function of your stomach.

After six months, you start weaning yourself off the medication for acid reflux, with the approval and guided support of the prescribing doctor.

You have alternatives for the foods that you love. They aren't the same, but for healing your stomach, you are willing to do it.

After another three months, you are off your medication. You keep taking the supplements for a few more months. And if you decide to continue with the foods that you used to eat all the time, but in limited quantity, you stay on the supplements to make sure you don't go back to what you had before.

A New Definition of Health

Research shows that if you don't fully understand a word and then read beyond it, your mind doesn't fully register anything that comes after it.

For that reason, some definitions of the individual words within the new definition of health are listed here.

To fully understand this, please do this:

1. Read the definition of health.

2. Look at the definitions of each word. The defined ones are in italics. Please look even if you know them, just to make sure you're looking at the correct definition of the word—as many have more than one meaning.

3. Then go back and reread the new definition of health.

The more you understand the definition, the more power you will have over your health. That means less suffering, less time at doctors' offices, and more time enjoying life.

> **Health occurs when an individual understands and *chooses* habits that strengthen, *restore,* and *enhance* their *organs, cells,* and *atoms* such that (disease and infirmity are conspicuously absent while) the *joy* of physical, mental, and social *vitality* are deliberately and reliably present.**

This definition takes the mystery out of understanding what health means, puts the understanding in, and gives you choice.

With this definition, YOU are responsible because you are to understand and choose the habits that will restore and enhance your health, all of which are explained—in a simple, easy-to-understand way—in the pages that follow.

Infirmity and disease are still absent. But in addition to this, your physical, mental, and social vitality are present, which means that they are included in the measurement of your health.

To make the process of working through this text easier for you and to make sure that you are milking everything you can out of the new definition of health, here are the individual words used and their relevant meanings.

They have been chosen carefully and deliberately. By being on the same page about what we are looking for in health, the rest of the book will make more sense to you. The power for being healthy is truly within your own hands.

Read the definitions, then go back and reread the new definition of health.

Choose

- Pick out or select (someone or something) as being the best or most appropriate of two or more alternatives; decide on a course of action, typically after rejecting alternatives. (Oxford Dictionary)

- To select freely and after consideration. (Merriam-Webster Dictionary)

For our purposes, you will look at options and consider them. You will choose freely based on your understanding of the alternatives.

Restore

- To repair or renovate so as to return it to its original condition. (Oxford Dictionary)

- To put or bring back into existence or use; to bring back to or put back into a former or original state. (Merriam-Webster Dictionary)

Obviously, you will not suddenly become twenty years younger, but there are supplement protocols developed and designed to jump-start organs as a car battery gets jump-started. This isn't treating disease; it's just helping an organ work so well that it is not hospitable to disease.

Enhance

- To intensify, increase, or further improve the quality, value, or extent of. (Oxford Dictionary)

- To increase or improve in value, quality, desirability, or attractiveness. (Merriam-Webster Dictionary)

Once an organ has been restored, the goal is to keep it at optimal functioning and of high quality of function. There will be more information about this in the following chapters.

Vitality

- The state of being strong and active; energy, the power giving continuance of life, present in all living things. (Oxford Dictionary)

- Lively and animated character, the power of enduring, the capacity to live and develop; physical and mental vigor especially when highly developed. (Merriam-Webster Dictionary)

Clearly, this would be an optimal way to go through life. I've gotten myself to this point. Lots of other people have as well. All of it is strategic and you will learn about it. You deserve to feel this great as well.

Joy

- A feeling of great pleasure and happiness; a thing that causes joy. (Oxford Dictionary)

- The emotion evoked by well-being, success, or good fortune or by the prospect of possessing what one desires; a state of happiness or felicity. (Merriam-Webster Dictionary)

When your body is functioning well and is out of pain, the natural state is one of joy. This is where the choices you make for your body give you access to a stronger and deeper experience of life, especially your spiritual life.

The following definitions are to clarify the parts of your body that you are caring for:

Organ

- A differentiated part of an organism, such as an eye, wing, or leaf, that performs a specific function. (Oxford Dictionary)

Cell

- The smallest structural unit of an organism that is capable of independent functioning, consisting of cytoplasm, usually one nucleus, and various other organelles, all surrounded by a semipermeable cell membrane. (Oxford Dictionary)

Atom

- The basic unit of a chemical element. (Oxford Dictionary)

I will go into more detail on the atom later in the book.

Here are some of the connections between your mental, physical, and social life and joy, including your spiritual life.

Mental vitality and joy: Being patient and kind with yourself, being appreciative of yourself—the beautiful and imperfectly perfect person you are, being able to grasp information, overcome challenges with kindness toward yourself and others, facing the day with hope and optimism—in spite of, and sometimes because of, the circumstances. And forgiving yourself as you learn to treat yourself with such kindness.

Physical vitality and joy: When you overcome challenges to your health, there is joy in being able to exercise or eat something that was once making you sick or knowing that your disease is regressing and that you'll be around for your grandkids or children. There is much to enjoy in our physical world.

Social vitality and joy: When you interact with those who lift you up and participate in organizations and movements that you believe make the world a better place. The people you surround yourself with strive to make the world a better place and are free of the conversations and activities that take away from vitality and joy. Social vitality also means that the conversations are loving and compassionate toward others who see the world differently than you.

Health is an interconnected web between what and how you think, what you feel, what you eat, and how you exercise.

In the following chapters, we will explore the different paradigms of health, and then we'll get into what you can do about getting to the good stuff.

2

How Healthy Can You Actually Become?

How much energy do you have? A lot? A little? Do you wake up tired? Do you wake up with energy, ready to go? Do you need drugs or medications so you can function at your best? Do you have trouble sleeping and wake up tired? Are you too tired to exercise? If you do exercise, is recovery long and painful?

These symptoms are all signs that your body isn't getting what it needs to operate. You can cover the problems with medications and stop feeling the discomfort—until more goes wrong. This manipulates your body and can enhance longevity, but not vitality.

Or you can give your body what it needs to operate and stop feeling the discomfort. This approach works with your body, enhancing both longevity and vitality.

Your body only has so much energy to spend. That energy is used to get you through the day, digest your food, repair organs while you're sleeping, keep your brain sharp, and more—to keep you healthy.

When you are not at your maximum, you need more sleep and rest because the energy that you do have has to be redirected to healing. The more natural energy your body generates through healthy and strategic means, the more it can be used to get you through the day and keep you functioning.

You can do much to increase your innate energy, and the task is less overwhelming if you have a strategic plan. My patients make this change every day.

Who You Get Your Advice From?

Pro tip: If you are trying to achieve a sustainable level of health with longevity thrown in, remember to take advice only from people in a position you'd like to be in or, at the very minimum, from someone who is at least one step ahead of you.

All the degrees and training in the world mean nothing if application and results haven't been achieved.

The more you give your body what it needs, the healthier and stronger you become. You will also only be as healthy as you believe and conceive you can be. If you look at the higher levels of health and think that's impossible, remember that the limitation starts in your mind.

If you get stuck in the thought of certain levels of health being impossible and you would like to move past it, but can't, then you'll want to work through my book *Visualization to Manifestation* or work with the EMBeR (Emotional & Mental Balancing & Repatterning) sessions to help you overcome that barrier to your goal. EMBeR is explained in my book *Intuition, Faith, and Freedom: The one at-home tool you need to avoid using medical intervention.*

Simply taking action can also change your mind.

Level 1: Managing Disease and Illness

Managing disease is where the majority of people view health. Health insurance pays for level 1 care. It is the most accepted level and is reinforced in media, advertising, news reports, and entertainment.

At this level, many people take one or more medications to avoid experiencing symptoms. Because they don't feel their symptoms, they are led to believe that they are healthy. This type of thinking goes back to the definition of health by the World Health Organization. People are experiencing physical, mental, and social well-being, which is managed with pharmaceutical drugs.

People operating at this level don't experience the body's subtle—yet significant—sensitivity to toxins. They either don't feel the effects, or they don't feel it to the degree that those at levels 2 and 3 feel it. They are largely disconnected from their bodies and their intuition as it relates to their health.

At this level, the energy in the body is going toward fighting off the chemicals and other interferences in the body, which will be explained later. The lifestyle advice is barely enough to give them a slight sense of power over their health. But it also gives them an out:

- "I know that I should eat better, but the medications are taking care of it. I'm fine. I can do what I want, and I feel great."

- "I know I should exercise/lose weight, but my test results are coming back better now that I'm taking these pills."

- "I don't really feel anything, but I can function throughout the day without getting depressed."

While on the medications, if these people are taking minimal if any action with their lifestyle choices (food, exercise, emotional health), the underlying problem will just continue getting worse.

If it does get better, it's a testament to the incredible healing ability and inclination for survival of the body.

The choices they are making have not addressed the cause of the underlying problem. It becomes obvious that this is also why, when someone starts a medication, they often have to stay on it.

At level 1, the energy of the body is focused on survival and managing illnesses. The emotional imprint for health at level 1 is anxiety, fear, anger, not caring, neglect, apathy, obsession (such as with food), the fight-flight-freeze response, frustration, blaming, unworthiness, despair, and antagonism.

The antagonism at this level becomes most obvious when they are presented with information outside what they can conceive as possible. This is where name-calling and judgment show up. It is not your job to change their mind. It is your job to accept where they are and love yourself enough to choose something kinder for your body's health.

Level 2: Healing Organs

At this level, there is some essential healing going on while medications may still be necessary. Health insurance pays for some level 2 care.

This is the level of healing that we see in modern medicine. You make small lifestyle changes, and you can keep your health at the level it is, or perhaps you can make some minor improvements.

The dietitian's recommendations have just enough information to help their patients maintain their level of illness or perhaps even get a little bit better. But the underlying assumption is that once you have a problem, it will be a problem forever. All decisions are made from this assumption.

You might take some supplements. Vitamin D, fish oil, and calcium are the most recommended supplements based on what my patients have reported. They receive just enough information to help keep them from getting worse quickly.

Many people are stuck in the belief that this is as good as health gets. The assumption is that as soon as you enter the disease process, there is no getting out of it, unless you cut out the organ or even replace it.

At level 2, the energy in the body is focused on the continual repair of the organs as the damage continues. There is some relief and improvement due to taking the supplements and making the small lifestyle changes.

People thinking at this level often eat organic foods and use essential oils, herbal supplements, and other natural remedies to address symptoms and diagnoses. However, they still believe that this is as good as it gets.

Many natural health providers also operate within this paradigm. These include muscle testing practitioners, functional medicine providers, and natural doctors.

The emotional imprint at this level is neutrality, contentment, boredom, courage, satisfaction, neutrality, and general trust. Because there is such contentment at this level and because they are doing better than most people they know, many patients don't look beyond this level.

Level 3: Restoring Organ Function

This is the level where your health improvements start getting interesting. This is when people's organs start working again, medications are dropping off, and disease processes are reversing. Health insurance does not pay for level 3 care. However, Health Share Plans often do.

Health Share Plans are sometimes called Health Care Sharing Ministries. Most offer faith-based membership committed to true prevention, like eating healthy foods, exercising, not smoking, not drinking in excess, and not using drugs.

Most people entering this level have something valuable they are in danger of losing (life or any hope of being pain/disease free) or something to live for (family, a God-given purpose) that has them stretching beyond level 2. They are willing to do whatever it takes to restore their organs.

This is the level where many people start living outside the box of the normal paradigm.

No one who gets to this level of health is merely treating disease. At this level of health, you are helping the body get stronger by supplying the organs with what they need to restore their function. At the low end of this level, some are still on medications as their bodies are beginning to work.

This is the domain of Nutrition Response Testing, one type of analysis I use with my patients. All advanced practitioners are trained in the restoration of organ function, although some are still operating at level 2.

Finding a medical doctor at this level is exceedingly rare, although they do exist. Remember how level 1 has the emotional imprint of antagonism? You will see the doctors in level 3 on the receiving end of antagonism. When you see antagonism directed at one of these doctors, there is an excellent chance the doctor has valuable wisdom to share.

In level 3, you are also supporting your body with nutrients through food and strategic supplementation to get as healthy as possible.

The body in the first two levels is dealing with many challenges that cause interference to its functioning. In the level 3 phase of healing, the interferences get addressed, reduced, and eliminated.

The interferences come from bugs, manmade materials, scars, and inner interference.

- Bug interference: bacteria, viruses, parasites, fungus

- Manmade interference: metals, chemicals, food sensitivities

- Scars: Scars interfere with nerve flow. This can be explained through an analogy. Imagine a lamp. The lamp is your organ. The cord going to the wall is the nerve going to the organ. If the cord is frayed, the lamp will flicker. When you put electrical tape on it, the lamp stops flickering and works. The lamp is your organ, the cord is your nerve, and the electrical tape is the treatment for the scar.

- Inner interference: mental stress, emotional stress, spiritual stress. These are most effectively addressed by releasing the neurologically imprinted energy and mental blocks and then creating new ones.

In my office, we mainly use Emotional & Mental Balancing & Repatterning (known as EMBeR). As the body is strategically supported in dealing with each of these interferences, it has more energy to direct to the operation of the organs rather than to deal with these interferences.

Once you get here, you are arriving at your innate state of health. At level 3, you have become excellent at identifying and eliminating the interferences. You know when something is off. This is the point where the body is starting to operate well without any medications.

This is where the immune system becomes strong and consistently reliable. This is where alternative therapies respond quickly in your body, and medications become largely unnecessary. Not only do medications become unnecessary, but you are so in tune with your body that you can sense or feel when they interfere with your body's functioning.

At this level, you are mindful of what you eat, drink, and think. You have done a certain level of inner work and have come to accept that you are operating on a different level than most people. You have the inner strength to be different from most other people. You have stopped trying to explain what you are doing and live by example.

How healthy you want to be will determine how much of a change you are willing to make. You know and accept this and make changes accordingly.

The emotional imprint of this level is reason, cheerfulness, hopeful, cautious, optimism, acceptance, and forgiveness; positive outcomes are expected.

Emotional Imprint and Invisible Waves

Before explaining the dynamics of level 4, it is important for you to have a basic idea of emotional imprints and invisible waves. You've heard of radio waves, 5G waves, sound waves. Brain waves. These are invisible but can be measured with special instruments.

You've likely heard of the increased breast cancer risk from women putting their cell phones in their bras. This is from invisible waves from the cell phone. You can't see them, and many people can't feel them—but they are there.

5G waves are damaging to the cells in our body. Some devices help lower them in your environment.

Music creates waves. There is a resonance of waves that supports healing. It is at the 432 Hz frequency. The more you have those waves in your environment, the better for you.

Emotions also create invisible waves. The waves emanating from love are coherent and create beautiful patterns, while those emanating from hate have the opposite effect. There is more on this in the section on atoms.

Level 4: Enhancing Organ Function

Enhancing organ function means taking the organs beyond the level of healing and moving them to optimum functioning. Like with level 3, health insurance does not pay for level 4 care. Health Share Plans often do.

You are vital, healthy, and milking the most out of life. Your emotions are balanced, and you feel fantastic. When you get off-kilter, you can get yourself back on quickly and easily.

Because of the inner work you have done, you are solidly planted in reality, and making healthy choices is the norm. Making unhealthy choices such as bingeing, overeating, overdrinking, putting toxins in your body, and exposing your mind to the influences of lower emotional imprints isn't an option for you.

That doesn't mean you don't ever expose yourself to such behaviors. It means you don't expose yourself to the degree that these behaviors harm you. Sometimes that means cutting something entirely out of your life. Sometimes it means just limiting a certain behavior.

You know what that line is because you are in tune with your body. And you wouldn't make choices that are unloving to you.

You know what the interferences are and avoid them as much as possible.

When an organ is functioning optimally, it does not need medications to work. At this level, the manmade medications become an obvious interference to your health and may even cause the body to drop down to as low as level 1.

You realize that most people reside at levels 1 and 2, so you get most of your health-enhancing information from those who have forged the path to level 4. Those entrenched at the lower levels exhibit their emotional imprint for that level, so rather than explain what you are doing, you live by example.

You confidently say no to medications, vaccinations, gossip, inflammatory news sources, and more. You find alternatives because you are operating on a different level. You focus on enhancing the function of the body, organs, cells, and atoms—you are not treating disease. You know that disease has no place in a body that has a strong foundation.

The emotional imprint of this level is enthusiasm, happiness, joy, love, gratitude, peace, faith, and eagerness.

It takes a level of discipline, faith, love, and mental toughness to get to the higher levels of health. This is simply because you are operating outside a system that most of the people in the world are living in. And they can't relate.

It is common for a patient who has gotten off medications and/or reversed a disease process to hear from their medical doctor: "I cannot recommend that. But whatever you are doing, keep doing it."

The patient is usually surprised that the medical doctor doesn't ask for more information. But the doctor is inside the box of medicine and has to stay there to maintain their license and keep working. Those of us at level 4, and sometimes level 3, are outside the box.

Keep in mind that there is a gradient of improvement for everyone. As life happens, you may travel up and down that gradient.

If you get to level 4 and are operating there and suddenly something traumatic or shocking happens out of left field, you may drop down to a lower level. An accident, loss of a job, loss of a family member, having to become a caretaker for a parent—all of these increase the stress that lowers levels of health.

The amount of time you drop depends on your mental toughness and discipline. Be honest with yourself but also kind. It does no good to beat yourself up.

If you lack discipline and mental toughness, completing the 75 Hard Program will help you (www.75hard.com).

Above all, be aware of where you are. Have grace for yourself and others. For yourself, also have the kind of love where you love yourself enough to not let yourself off the hook.

The Learning Process

You will likely be learning a lot of helpful new concepts and information. There is a learning curve. The goal is to get to consciously competent and unconsciously competent. These are the levels of learning and awareness.

Everyone goes through these levels as they learn. So use this as a way to understand where you are on the spectrum. The more you expose yourself to the information and implement what you are learning, the higher up the ladder you will go.

Unconsciously incompetent: You find the information in this book interesting but have little to no idea what I am talking about. You are likely at level 1.

Here's an analogy: A child doesn't even know what a tricycle is. Maybe it has just been introduced as a possibility of something to do. She has seen others on a bicycle and doesn't even think of it as a possibility for herself. It's something the big kids do.

Consciously incompetent: You are aware of where you are lacking skills and are working on learning them. You may get frustrated sometimes. For the most part, you are successfully failing. This means that you make mistakes, but you are trying. The more you put yourself in a situation that stretches you enough to fail, the more you learn.

Here, the child has mastered the tricycle. She sees the big kids on the bicycle and knows it is a possibility. Dad got her a bicycle. She has given it a try but has a hard time. Dad has to hold onto the back of the bike. When he lets go, she tips over.

Consciously competent: You have failed so many times in being consciously incompetent that you are now consciously competent. You have landed at the next level.

The child in our example can stay up on the bicycle, but the front of the bicycle is shaky. She doesn't quite have the pedaling down; the front shakes back and forth as she tries to hold on. She started by tipping over, but now she is starting to be able to put on the brakes. As long as she thinks about it, she can do it.

Unconsciously competent: You don't have to think about it. For example, when you become consciously competent at what you need to do to keep your health at level 2, you may be consciously incompetent at level 3. As you become more skilled at what it takes to have your health be at level 3, you become consciously competent.

When you become unconsciously competent at level 3, you may naturally move up to level 4.

For the girl on the bicycle, she doesn't have to think about it. Only when she is on different terrain. But she understands her bike well enough that she can navigate just about anything. And flying down those hills sure is fun.

3

Your Body Has a Mind of Its Own

Has this ever happened to you?

You tell yourself: "I am not going to eat sugar today." You go to work. Someone sets out a plate of cookies, donuts, or a birthday cake. You remember your resolve. The next thing you know, you look down, and half a plate of cake is in your mouth, and you don't even know how it happened.

Your body took over. You say "screw it" and continue to eat, breaking your promise to yourself—yet again. And then you get to deal with all the emotions of disappointment that go along with it.

We have all been there.

What happens in this situation is that your body-mind has taken over. Your body's job is to keep you alive and as engaged in life as possible. It will do what it thinks is best, based on how you have trained it, regardless of what you think.

For most of us, we have given over our connection to our body and what it needs to others. We look outside ourselves for answers and are influenced by outside influences—advertisements, news shows, magazine articles, social media. It is socially acceptable and even encouraged to treat our bodies in a way that is indulgent and unhealthy.

Your connection with your body is your gut instinct. Your gut instinct is a gateway to understanding and helping your body with what it needs to be healthy. With your children, it shows up as a mother's intuition.

As we have been encouraged to trust the science or trust the news or trust the politicians or trust the doctor more than you trust your gut or trust yourself or trust your mother's intuition, the disconnect has become bigger and bigger. And, unfortunately, normalized.

Now is the time for you to reconnect with your body *and* be in charge of your health. The more you pay attention to your gut instinct, the more your body's innate wisdom begins to reveal itself to you. This type of connection with your body is part of your human instinct and nature.

You see it in newborns who instinctively know to seek out food from their mother's breast as soon as they are born. You had it when you were born, so you can reconnect with it. Once this communication with your body reconnects, the wisdom your body reveals to you becomes obvious and easy.

All you have to do is start paying attention to your body's messages and you will relearn it.

You Are Not Your Body—Your Body Is Not You

Many people think that they are interchangeable with their bodies. But you are not your body. There is the *you* that is the spiritual being. And then there is *your body*.

The pineal gland connects the spiritual and the physical. It is the access point to experiencing God. The pineal gland is found in medical imaging by looking for calcification around it. This calcification is made of fluoride. Fluoride is added to our water, vaccines, toothpaste, and more.

During the detoxification process of your journey toward health, metals will be released from your body, including your brain. The more you support your body against the constant bombardment of toxins and the more you support your health, the greater your connection with God. If you think you have a great connection now and you are not at level 4 health, just wait.

You (spiritual being) are the custodian of your body. Merriam-Webster defines a custodian as one that guards and protects or maintains. Your body is attached to your thoughts, decisions, and everything else, so it is not going anywhere. It is dependent on you for your care of it.

The state of health of your body is a direct reflection of how much of the custodian role you have taken on. For this reason, no one outside of you deserves to be trusted with that care unless they have proven themselves.

At level 1, just because someone has a medical degree, that's not enough to trust them. At level 2, a medical degree with evidence of competence is required to trust them. At level 3, you start looking for outside-the-box evidence.

When your body has taken over, it is because it has been indulged, not trained, and it has learned not to trust you. Your body acts and responds a lot like a six-year-old child.

I confidently say this because I spent a few years as a first-grade teacher. Like our bodies, the children at this age are caught somewhere between the spiritual world and life here on earth. They are searching for clear boundaries, safety, security, and fairness.

When they have these qualities, they go forth confidently throughout their day. When they don't have these assurances, they act out.

When the rules continually change, like with fad diets that you change every three to six months, the body gets confused and acts out. Changing diets all the time and inconsistent eating patterns often lead to binge eating and regretful choices, like that piece of candy or the cake at the office.

When the rules are clear and are kept, a child will remain enthusiastic and calm. The same is true for your body. Consistent food quality, quantity, and eating patterns keep your body calm. It is also kind and loving to yourself to do this.

It is most often the case that when you have binged, your body has not been sufficiently fed with nutrients. This leads to more cravings and more acting out on the part of your body.

When dealing with a six-year-old, if acknowledgment is pointed out and given for good behavior, she feels good, and that behavior continues. You might say to her, "I see that you helped Andrea with putting the blocks away. That was very kind of you. You did a good job."

Noticing and acknowledging yourself for choosing the carrots over the carrot cake creates a feeling of security and trust in your body—and, if your body is given enough food, it's less likely to binge.

If a child is reprimanded with anger for pulling someone's hair, the child will respond by stomping around and being angry.

Telling yourself you failed again and giving yourself messages such as "look how bad you are for having some cake" don't work. Then you get mad at yourself and decide to eat two cakes because, forget it, you messed up, so why not.

But if you respond to the child with firm kindness and hold her to account with something more along the lines of, "That was not very kind of you. And I know you are a kind person.

You hurt the child whose hair you pulled. Let's apologize," then the child is more likely to behave kindly.

Acknowledge to yourself that you ate a piece of cake even though you said you wouldn't. Then check in with yourself to find out why.

- Had you not eaten enough of the healthy food before being in the room with the cake?

- Had you not been clear to yourself that you wouldn't eat it?

- Were you feeling guilty and valuing someone else's opinion over your health?

- Was someone unkind to you, and was your reaction to be unkind to yourself as well, instead of setting a healthy boundary?

- What did you need to do to care for yourself that had you make that choice?

- Was that kind and loving to you?

These are the reflections that people go through as they figure it out. When you figure out what your reaction is, you can fix it. If you don't explore your reaction, the behaviors will come back time and time again.

I caution you, however, in overdoing the analysis. You can get caught up in analyzing and never get the result. This is a form of indulgence and keeps you feeling safe but doesn't support your health. This is where discipline comes into play.

For some people, discipline isn't accessible. In this case, there may be emotional blocks that keep you stuck. There may be mental habits that keep you stuck.

Many people make the mistake of thinking that they are doing something wrong. If you are that person, let me assure you, you are not. Your emotions or mental habits are stuck in a neurological pattern. Neurological patterns can be interrupted by discipline. However, if you don't have a habit of discipline, many techniques are available to support you.

I spent years using and getting trained in many techniques including Emotional Freedom Technique, Psych-K, Emotion Code, meditation, prayer, and more to help unstick my patterns. Over time I developed a new, usable technique that is so simple you can take it with you anywhere and use it any time: EMBeR: Emotional & Mental Balancing & Repatterning.

These are all options for changing your mental and emotional patterns. If you have been struggling for months or years with an issue, I encourage you to look into them.

Setting Yourself Up to Not Have Cravings

The way to set yourself up to not have cravings was something I saw in my first-grade classroom when I had started my health restoration journey.

We all know sugar makes kids crazy. I was alone with twenty-five first graders. Twenty-five first graders on sugar were more than any one teacher should have to deal with. So whenever there were classroom parties, which were usually sugar-fests with cupcakes and other treats, I started doing Fancy Five Course Parties instead.

I had learned enough about food to realize that I could avoid the sugar high of twenty-five six-year-olds if I got other food in them instead. It worked much better than I expected. By the time we got to course 5, they had no appetite left.

I decided to implement this plan in my personal life as well. It has worked well for me, and I expect it will work well for you too.

Basically, when you eat, you go down this list.

If you still crave something by course 5, go ahead and have some kind of treat. Ideally, it'll be a healthy one. But sometimes fruit will take care of it.

As you learn the healthier options, this becomes less of a problem for your health, and it's still enjoyable. If you've loaded up on the items higher on the list, you often won't crave the last by the time you get there.

Course 1: Healthy, fresh vegetables

Course 2: Healthy meats (since these are eaten as a close second, the high-quality fats here break down the fat-soluble nutrients in the vegetables)

Course 3: Fresh fruit

Course 4: Crackers

Course 5: Desserts

By the time you get to course 5, your body is often satisfied and feeling healthy. Maybe you just give yourself a bite of something. Often, you may not want a donut or a candy at all.

The trick is having those vegetables on hand. If you don't have time to food prep, then get the veggies that are prepped for you at the grocery store. (Yes, we should all prepare, but there is a reality about time that 99 percent of people haven't conquered.)

If you just start with this, you will get much healthier.

Your body, like a six-year-old's, will be calmer and happier and will respond better to the surprises that life dishes out.

Since YOU are the custodian of your body, you ultimately make the decisions and are responsible for the care of YOUR BODY. As your body learns to trust that it will not be starved, it will act out less. If it is sure of when it will get meals or that it will get enough food to supply the organs with much-needed nutrients, it will no longer grab whatever is in front of it and eat.

Your body will make the best decisions it can, but its decisions are based on its experience as a knee-jerk reaction. Like a six-year-old, your body needs structure and needs to know what it can count on. If it is in a state of survival (which most bodies are when starting this journey), your body will take over and have you perform unintended behaviors like stuffing your face with cake.

Don't get mad at yourself (or if you do, forgive yourself as quickly as possible). Just notice what you've done and realize that you probably didn't give your body enough healthy food. The chapter on healthy food will give you some guidance on what that means.

The body feels unsafe when it is given experiences that take away from its health. The body feels safe when given experiences that enhance its health.

How to Keep Your Body Feeling Safe and Loved

Experiences that cause the body to feel safe and be healthy are these:

- Foods free of toxins and chemicals often labeled *organic* or *sustainably raised* (The word *natural* on foods is largely unregulated and a marketing ploy.)

- Environments free of toxins and chemicals

- Expanding the exposure to the higher frequencies and vibrations such as love (528 Hz) or gratitude (432 Hz), most easily found with music

- Movement and exercise, including those that get the heart rate up—stretching, running, jumping

- Sufficient rest, which varies from person to person

- Clear structure on what the body can expect

Experiences that cause the body to be stressed enough to be unhealthy are these:

- Toxins and chemicals in the food, water, and air

- Exposure to the lower frequencies such as worry, fear, anxiety, hate

- Mental exposure to conversations, literature, and media input filled with fear, anxiety, grief, anger, hate

- Eating dead foods (such as many packaged and processed foods—just because it says on the label that it's healthy doesn't mean that it's healthy)

- Avoiding exercise or only doing minimal exercises. Walking 10,000 steps is the start of great health and an important, valid step for many. Having such exercise be the end goal will keep you at level 1 health.

- Chaotic eating or lots of changes in diet and schedules, including not giving yourself enough calories

When you start to consistently make the health-giving choices for your body, your body will likely rebel. It will have sugar cravings as it seeks the familiar. It will also start getting healthy (and behave) for you, especially as you become more consistent with what you give it. If you try to do these changes all at once, it will freak your body out. So don't.

You will learn about all the suggestions here, but start with the one thing that you think will be easiest for you to take charge of.

There are four categories. Pick one of them. Then, choose a specific action that is simple enough for you to just do. If you've been on this path for a while, stretch yourself and do as many as you can or choose something to improve yourself a little more.

1. Choose healthier food.

    a. Choose one organic or sustainably raised vegetable over the regular ones. Pick one vegetable.

    b. Eat a vegetable every day. Pick one you feel comfortable eating.

    c. Other_____

2. Expose yourself to higher frequencies.

    a. Stop watching the news every night and instead watch a show from a church or on meditation or about people helping people.

    b. Read religious or spiritual text (such as the Bible) for ten minutes a day.

    c. Other_____

3. Exercise daily.

    a. Choose an exercise program and start it.

    b. Figure out why you are not exercising and take care of it. If you have inadequate shoes, buy some. If you are embarrassed or uncomfortable at the gym, exercise at home instead. If you pick an exercise that you don't like or is too hard or too easy, then change it. Pick a program that's at your level.

    c. Go for a walk or learn how to jog safely.

    d. Other_____

4. Avoid toxins.

    a. Go to Environmental Working Group (www.EWG.org) to learn about toxins in your products so you can make another choice.

    b. Pick a product for your lotion that is paraben-free.

    c. Get a water filter for your house. (One is better than none, and Berkey is better than most—do what's best for you.)

    d. Other_____

Now, let's dig into some basics of how a healthy body works and what you can do to help yours.

4

Organs, Cells, and Atoms (but mostly atoms)

Atoms make up the cells in your body, the cells make up the organs, the organs make up the organ systems, and the organ systems make up your entire body.

Having a basic understanding of what is happening with the atoms in your body is helpful for when you make choices in your life, simply because you will have a greater understanding of how they affect your health.

If you have taken any human biology classes, then you have studied the organs and the cells in some way. Most references to health, even alternative health, is directed at the body's organs, organ systems, and cells. None of my medical classes addressed atoms and how those relate to health.

Fortunately, a much-needed shift is taking place where a handful of scientists are looking at atoms, how they are broken down, how they are affected, and how that affects health. As we get into the more subtle aspects of what affects health, the effects of your daily choices will become more apparent to you.

Atoms

Atoms are made of 99.999999999 (and so on)% energy. This means that they are mostly space. This space is affected by the waves that we cannot see. We can, however, feel them. If you can't feel atoms yet, then you need to know that they are there. You will gain a sense of atoms over time.

This might show up by looking at a table of food options at a potluck and feeling what some of the foods will do to your body if you eat them.

We innately can sense these invisible waves of energy, but modern life has trained us away from this ability. Fortunately, you can relearn it.

Emotional Waves

The emotional waves are where the rubber meets the road in regard to health. The emotional waves affect your atoms, so are foundational to your health. This is something fundamental that gets ignored or not written about because it's too hippy-dippy or out there. Or people think it's a nice concept, but they don't know what to do about it.

I care about results, and certain energies cause damage, and other energies cause healing. This is why you can do all the right things and still be sick, still have the pain and physical limitations, still have the anxiety, still have cancer, and still not be getting better.

I've had two spontaneous healings because I implemented this information. All the diet and therapy in the world didn't help me. It got me to a certain point where I could manage the pain and discomfort. But that was it.

I meditated for two to four hours every day for months, as taught by Dr. Joe Dispenza. The healings occurred during two separate retreats. The first healing was from gripping anxiety that was released. The second was getting movement back in my left hip.

Because of these spontaneous healings, I have been able to exercise without pain since late 2019. I now bring love and gratitude to every exercise I do because the emotional waves of love and gratitude facilitate healing. And I plan to keep my body able to move as it does.

When someone says that everything you need is right inside of you, it is true. If you feel hateful or angry, or victimized by someone, these are lower emotional waves. They will keep you sick.

Have you ever stood next to a furious or significantly troubled person? Did you feel it? Those were waves. Have you ever been around a person who radiated love—and all you wanted to do was sit in their presence? That person is emitting waves of love.

These waves affect your body at the level of your atoms. The more you expose yourself to love and gratitude throughout your day, the more your body will move toward health.

Messages from Water

In his book *Hidden Messages from Water*, Dr. Masaru Emoto uses high-speed photography to show that crystals found in frozen water become beautiful, bright-colored snowflake patterns when exposed to loving words. The water crystals become asymmetrical patterns with dull colors when exposed to pollution or unkind words.

Your body is made of up to 60 percent water. What do you think the words you say and the energy you surround yourself with means for your body and your health?

The more you expose yourself to anger, fear, and worry during the day, the more challenge you are giving your body in moving toward health. If you do not have a say in your anxiety, anger, or depression, then there are options for getting control of them. Remember, this is an energetic conversation, not a psychological one. We are focusing on the energy here, not on the psychological analysis of it.

There is no failure or shame in starting with where you are. The only actual failure is not taking the first step, giving up, and not trying again.

We are bombarded daily with worry, fear, anger—the drama of the news, the worry about our futures. Just become aware of these emotions and start looking at the options for what you can change.

You may be addicted to these lower emotions. You know you are when you can't turn them off or when you find yourself leaving them in one scenario, like a job, and noticing them showing up in another, like a new relationship.

Wean yourself or go cold turkey. Learn how to release them with EMBeR (Emotional & Mental Balancing & Repatterning). How you take care of them, that's up to you. Just play with it and figure out what works for you.

Keep in mind that emotions do affect organs. For example, anger is linked to liver problems, worry is linked to stomach problems, and fear is linked to kidney problems.

The simplest way to start making the shift in your energy is to start with five minutes of meditation a day. If you have a spiritual practice or belief, start heading in that direction. If you don't have one, just start with getting still for five minutes, and as you notice your mind wandering, give yourself kudos, credit, and a lot of appreciation for taking this step.

The emotions within a healthy body are *mainly* focused on love, joy, and gratitude.

What Is a Good Meditation?

Pro tip: On meditation: People have the mistaken belief that a good meditation is one where your mind doesn't wander. This is false. A good meditation is one where you catch your mind wandering and bring it back to the present moment. Every time you notice your mind wander, you have been successful at your meditation.

Notice I wrote *mainly*. This is because you are human, and sometimes other emotions come up and are present.

When you hold other feelings within yourself, reinforced by not only your thoughts but what you voice about others or yourself, the practice reinforces a discordant pattern in your energy field. It is the discord that supports illness. This is why the practice of catching your thoughts and directing them to being present is so powerful in the process of healing.

Your habitual thoughts reinforce your feelings and also create thought patterns in your nervous system. Your nervous system is made up of cells called neurons. Neurons transmit chemical and electrical signals throughout your body. They do this by lining up with each other to transmit their messages, with the brain being the center of this communication. It is like the electrical system behind the walls in your house, but far more complex. Even more complex than a smart house.

Just like the electrical system in your house, you can't see your internal electrical system, but you can see its effects by how well the system is working. In your house, you know the electrical system works when your lights and appliances work. In your body, you know the nervous system works when your muscles, joints, and organs work. Your thoughts and thought patterns can consciously direct and change your nervous system.

So you can change the habitual thought patterns that have been making you sick. The thought patterns that make you sick are the ones that are opposite to the level of love, joy, and gratitude.

If you are practicing a few minutes a day in taking your thoughts from wandering and shifting them to being present or being focused on something spiritual, you are placing new neuron patterns in your brain. As these patterns get stronger, you will find that when you get in a situation where something goes wrong, you start noticing your emotions, seeing what happens, and then shifting them.

A major victory for most people is when you are faced with a familiar trigger, you notice your habitual reaction, stop it while it is happening, and choose a different response. You can then even get to where you look at the bad thing that happened and realize why it happened and how it might be contributing to your strengths and wisdom today.

Here is a simple example from my life. I had gone grocery shopping and had the groceries in my trunk. I parked the car in my garage, went to the back, and began taking them out.

One thing I enjoy doing since I've gotten stronger and healthier is loading up all my groceries in my arms and carrying them into the house in one load. (Simply because I can.) This includes going up a flight of stairs to get to the kitchen.

I generally just put one bag at a time on my left forearm. I reach in with my right hand and put it on my left arm. There were only a couple of bags left. I picked one up with my right hand and went to place it on my left forearm. The weight in the bag shifted.

Then I heard a crash. I stopped for a second. "Uh oh." What was that?

I looked down, and there on the cement was a big gooey mess of maple syrup with shards of glass in and around it. I observed what happened in my body and my mind. My heart clenched for a moment. The thoughts that would lead to drama and distress started running through my mind.

I noticed thought patterns of wasted money and food starting, but they never came to a full thought pattern or fixation or repetition. I have trained my mind. I stopped the thought patterns that wanted to come forth and shifted them to what needed to be done.

None of those originally trained thought patterns would help the situation. They would cause my body to feel a high level of stress (unhealthy). They could have, at another time, ruined my night. I could deal with the situation in a state of agitation or a state of indifference or a state of love and patience.

The large bottle of maple syrup had been carefully double bagged. I looked at the bag and saw the interesting way it was twisted so that the bottle could fall out.

There were facts. The fact was that there was broken glass and maple syrup on the ground. I chose to deal with it in a state of love and patience. I reassessed what I needed to do and what would be best.

It was dark out, and there was a lot of glass. The loving thing to do would be to clean up the mess right away, but since my garage is in an older house and does not have the best lighting, doing the clean-up in the light of day would be the more loving choice.

If I had been in a state of agitation, I may have been careless and perhaps would have tried cleaning it up without a glove barrier because I'd be trying to get it done quickly, and I would likely have injured myself.

I left the mess in the garage to clean up the next morning. It's something I could plan for. And the only possible disaster would be the attraction of bugs. But my safety and care are more important.

This is part of why my health is excellent. I meet myself and even my simplest challenges, as much as possible, with loving kindness. Berating and judging myself isn't a loving way to be toward myself. Just like berating and judging yourself isn't a loving way to be toward yourself.

Be aware of emotional suppression as well. Some people use meditation or prayer as a way to escape reality and suppress their negative emotions more. If you suppress your emotions, you might tell yourself that it's okay but still be in an agitated, hyper state. You tell yourself one thing while emotionally you don't believe the words you're telling yourself.

Emotion is what the body responds to.

Life is too precious to go around miserable, dramatic, or agitated all the time. You can get to know your thoughts to release them in two ways: by consciously shifting the emotion or by becoming aware of and consciously shifting your thought. They are the two sides of the coin.

By getting honest with yourself, giving yourself a boatload of love and compassion for that pain, and being able to count on yourself and trust yourself, these lower emotions release and get unstuck within you.

Until you face them off, they are in control. And once you've done it enough, you realize the relief and freedom on the other side of it, so you look for anything to let go of.

This isn't feel-good or soft and fluffy. It's raw, often ugly, and for many people there are a lot of tears. But it's also practical.

And freeing. Fortunately, and ironically, after you go through it, there's a level of peace that you can only know once you get there.

If you have trouble visualizing a different reality, how to do so is addressed in my book *Visualization to Manifestation.* The workbook companion walks you through some processes that also help you gently and caringly face and release some of the stuff that is keeping you feeling those negative vibes.

If you have trouble keeping your word to yourself, then doing Emotional & Mental Balancing & Repatterning (EMBeR) can help. The exercises in the visualization workbook also help.

Ultimately, getting your health to where you want it to be is up to you.

Some waves of energy emit from the emotions of anger, despair, longing, wanting, love, joy, happiness, appreciation, and gratitude. They can come from within you, as could have happened with the maple syrup, or from the environment around you.

Energy of Things Around You

As we are going down this path of waves and things, there is something to consider. But first, I will tell you a story from my distant past. It's about the energy around you.

I was a German major in the late 1980s and early 1990s. I studied the language and was fascinated by World War II. I was interested in the people: How did this happen? What was going on in their minds? In their lives? The wall between East and West Germany had come down the year before.

There was an opportunity to volunteer at a concentration camp memorial on the eastern side. The camp site had been closed since the war decades before. There was only one group who had been in it since then. I would be part of the second group, made up of volunteers in their late teens and early twenties.

East Germany was beautiful and untouched. It looked like it was still the 1940s and was fascinating to step into. We stayed in an old palace, which was surprisingly small. I was used to the Disney renditions. It was more like one of our large houses in the US today. But the landscape was stunning. It was fresh and clean.

At the concentration camp memorial, there were no buildings left, just their foundations. The foundations were covered with almost fifty years of plant overgrowth. Standing back and looking at it, you would have no idea that it had been a concentration camp. Our job was to find the foundations and remove the overgrowth so the layout of the camp would be easy to identify.

After a week of being together day and night, I needed some space. I decided to walk around and explore the foundations some more. The woods were beautiful, so I walked into them.

As I was walking, I started feeling pressure in my chest. I was confused about this. The farther I walked, the worse it got. At one point, I started gasping for air, panicked, and ran back to the group.

What was that?

I was shaking by the time I got back. I told the others about my weird experience, and we decided to walk back to the area together. We walked toward the area, and as we got closer, others started noticing the strange feeling. Just like me, they stopped at the point where I had turned and ran back.

We stood at that invisible wall and wondered what it was and what had happened there. It felt sinister. We rode our bikes back to the palace, sobered by our speculations of what could have happened, and decided not to venture to that area again.

The following week, we met a survivor at the camp. We told him what we had experienced and asked him if he knew what had happened there. He solemnly nodded, then confidently walked us to the area we had been the week before. He pointed to an imprint in the land where a series of horrific events occurred. It was clear why the wall of energy was there. But it is too horrible a story to tell here.

We each had a physical and appropriate response to the energy of the land. He knew what we were talking about because of how we had felt.

The point of the story is that your environment matters. Your body is picking up information from the environment that you can't see with your mind. The vibes that we felt in Germany was a huge and an obvious one.

The Gift of Boredom

Pro tip: When you are used to the emotions of fear, anxiety, anger (and others), shifting up to the higher levels requires that you move through boredom. You will often feel bored before you get to the feelings of relief, peace, and joy. So when you feel bored, keep going. You're on your way to joy.

Where you are matters. Who you surround yourself with matters. What you listen to matters. What you read or watch matters.

There are imprints of energy everywhere: in your environment, on your TV, on your radio, in your food. There are many steps along the way.

The imprint from Germany had been there for almost fifty years when we experienced it. Becoming aware of and managing the energy surrounding you is where people who are achieving and experiencing ever-improving and excellent health begin to look at and become selective with their environments, their conversations, and their foods.

Choose yours based on what you want to have in your life. It's essential to be selective (not obsessive) about your environment.

Part II

The 3 Contributors to Health That You Can Control

5

Healthy Stuff to Put in Your Body

Many different food lists and diets are available in the world. You've probably tried at least one or two or more of them. Jumping from diet to diet and fad to fad will confuse the body and put it more out of control, put it in a situation where it is likely to binge, and diets just won't work.

Before moving on, let's address a common misconception about being healthy and being fit. Most people collapse these two concepts and believe they are the same. They are not.

Being fit is important in enjoying life. It means that your muscles are strong and perhaps even defined. You are able to lift heavy objects, jog, and run. When you age as a fit person, you are not plagued with being unable to perform tasks such as lifting grandchildren, running a 5K or marathon, hiking, and kayaking.

One example of being fit and unhealthy is the example of a person who runs marathons. Carb-loading is what a person does the day before a marathon to give the body an extra boost of energy the next day.

An unhealthy, fit person will carb-load by eating regular ice cream, regular brownies, and French fries.

The healthy, fit person will carb-load by eating more fruit, sweet potatoes, real sourdough bread, and perhaps a homemade treat made with fruit and honey or maple syrup.

The unhealthy, fit person is putting junk in their bodies and foods that significantly increase inflammation and put strain on the heart and other organs.

The healthy, fit person will eat foods that are high-carb and yet mostly filled with nutrients and will focus on foods that do not increase inflammation but support the body's functioning.

We've all heard of the person who performs an intense activity, like a marathon or bike race, then collapses at the end with a heart attack. This is met with disbelief by those who have equated the ideas of fit and healthy. That person may be fit, but that person is not healthy.

A fit body can perform athletically. If that body is fed on refeed or carb-loading days with lots of sugar foods, it's not a healthy body. If they are full of anger or other lower emotions, they are fit, but not healthy.

To rein it in and create a level of stability for the body, it is important to give it the foundation of what bodies need: healthy, real foods. And love. (But this section is about the foods.)

A similar misconception occurs with the concept of being slender and healthy. It is assumed that a slender person is healthy. The thin person may be managing her hunger with cigarettes. Or she might be eating all diet, packaged foods that are full of preservatives and other chemicals. She may be thin, but she is not healthy.

As you move forward in improving your health, always keep in mind your specific needs. This is especially important if you have a diagnosed disease or disorder. There are suggested diets for most health issues. It is your responsibility to become an expert in the diet best for your condition.

People have had excellent results by combining the dietary recommendations for their own health condition and the recommendations here. For example, people with kidney disease are usually high in potassium. A lot of recommended foods for optimizing health are high in potassium. If you have kidney disease—or are headed that way—many of the recommended foods would not work for you.

If this is you, you'll look at the list of foods with low potassium that also qualify as healthy, by these standards here, and keep to that list.

The body doesn't lie. You can't cheat it, you can't trick it, you can't manipulate it, and be healthy.

Just to state the message once again: Jumping from diet to diet puts the body in a state of confusion. It gets confused and doesn't behave like you want it to. When you get plenty of quality foods, you are more focused and attentive, and you are less depressed, emotional, or reactive.

The foods your body needs to function well are quite basic. Your trained reaction might be to try and dodge, avoid, or tweak them. An example is this: If I just add a little sugar to it, that'll be okay. It's not. Adding sugar may cause your body to act out. And your body may act out as it is trying to figure out how serious you are about eating healthy foods.

Acting out in the case of your body includes anything that doesn't end up having you feel good. It could include binge eating, skipping exercise—just making choices that aren't nurturing to you. You haven't earned your body's trust.

You can expect your body to respond this way for about six weeks if you are consistent. If you are in terrible health and are desperate to get healthy, that motivation can cause it to change quickly. But for most people, change takes about six weeks.

The simplest way to start making the shift is by increasing quality foods while decreasing the others.

Quality of Foods

Quality foods are real foods. They have been taken from the ground or fed from the ground and are not interfered with by a human, except to wash or prepare for consumption. They have not been tampered with, not even with spices.

Vegetables, Grains, and Nuts: The best foods in this group are local organic or sustainably raised. (Small farms often can't afford the high price and a large amount of paperwork necessary to get the designation of organic but would be considered to be sustainably raised.)

The next best is local. The chemicals can be detoxified. Local foods tend to have more of the nutrients you need for the environment in which you live. An example of this is local honey, which is commonly used to help against seasonal allergies. The bees use the local flora, and their honey is known to help local people with their allergies. This philosophy can be transferred to all local food sources.

The next best is organic, nonlocal. Often these fields are downwind of a regular farm. They are still better than the ones that are full-on sprayed with chemicals.

Frozen organic would be next on your list. You're right that it isn't fresh, but it will have fewer chemicals and still includes nutrients.

The last choice would be your regular, run-of-the-mill grocery foods.

Fun Fact: Leafy green vegetables help pull toxins out of your body.

Fruits: Fruits follow the same rules as vegetables with a slight variation. If you eat its skin, it's best to have unsprayed foods. This is especially true for berries. Raspberries, strawberries, and blackberries are covered with tiny crevices that are virtually impossible to wash the pesticides and herbicides out of.

Foods that you peel are the better option.

Since fruits are likely genetically modified, you'll need to support your body's detoxification process. That isn't ideal but it's still so much better for you than other treats—like a regular candy bar.

Proteins: Vegetarianism has been more popular lately due to some movies educating people on how bad the meat industry is.

Most of the people taking on this new way of eating are dumping their fast-food habits. That in and of itself, due to the increase in vital nutrients and the substantial decrease in food additives and toxins, will improve health when you consider the improved quality of the food and the reduction in added chemicals.

The long-term problem with this is that your body needs essential amino acids. It also needs fats, which is addressed in the next section. When food is *essential*, that means that it needs to come from an outside source. The best, most available source of amino acids is from animal products.

The most important time to eat protein: breakfast.

Healing Specific Organs and Food

Fun fact: If you want to heal an organ, eat the organ or take a supplement with the organ in it. So to heal your liver, you eat liver. Many years ago in the US, and still today in other parts of the world, all parts of animals were eaten. Now we mainly only eat the muscles in the form of different cuts of meat. Organ meats are important for enhancing and sustaining health and are available in supplement form today.

Fats: We need fats. We also need the cholesterol in the fat from animal products. The one fact that I find striking is that we have been educated on the importance of having low-fat diets.

We have also had an increase in neurological issues in our society. The neurological issues include depression, anxiety, and Parkinson's.

You have probably heard of essential fatty acids (EFAs). It is often taken as a fish oil supplement and is one of the most recommended supplements by medical doctors. There is information on the different ratios of the different types of omegas; however, it's important to not get caught in the weeds of information.

What you need to know is that not having enough omega-3s creates inflammation and stiffness in your cell walls, which limits the movement of neurotransmitters and hormones throughout your body. What this means for you is that your stiff cells are likely the foundational problem in heart problems, cognitive problems, hormone problems, eye problems, and just your overall health.

Grain-fed animals, which is most animal meat found in stores today, don't have enough omega-3 fatty acids. They have plenty of omega-6 fatty acids. So eating grain-fed animals contributes to the inflammation and lack of cell pliability in your body.

Grass-fed animals have plenty of omega-3 fatty acids so they have an anti-inflammatory effect on your body.

Animal fats help prevent both depression and neurological issues. Like with everything, you need to consider the source of your fat. Toxins are stored in fats. If you eat animals that are given antibiotics and are fed foods sprayed with chemicals, those items can be stored in the fat.

The closer to nature and purer your source of foods, the fewer foods you will need to detoxify your body.

Best Food Choice Tip

Pro tip: The closer you are to the source of where the food originates (grown or raised), the healthier for you.

Food List Rules

The following food list is a baseline to start.

Never eat something on the list if you know you are sensitive to it. Don't eat items on the list if you are dealing with a disease that your special diet recommends against.

You can't cheat the system, fake the system, or take shortcuts while restoring your health. If you have bowel issues, skip the wheat (one possible exception being real sourdough), beans, and dairy, and be sure to cook the scrapy vegetables.

Scrapy vegetables (to be cooked—steamed, lightly sautéed, or baked) are those that scrape or tear you up anywhere from your esophagus (the tube from your mouth to your stomach) to your colon. If you have any irritation in any of these areas, pay close attention to this section. If you are uncertain if a food is scrapy, just put it between your hands and rub it together hard. If it's even a tiny bit rough, it may cause a problem inside of you.

Food List

Vegetables

(leaning toward scrapy, so best steamed or cooked)

Asparagus

Bamboo

Beans, green

Beet greens

Broccoli

Brussels sprouts

Cabbage

Cauliflower

Collard greens

Kale

Mustard greens

Pumpkin

Spinach

Squash (summer or zucchini)

Swiss chard

Turnips

Turnip greens

Vegetables

(okay to eat raw)

Celery

Cucumber

Fennel bulb

Hearts of palm

Jicama

Kimchee (don't eat if sensitive stomach)

Lettuces: arugula, butterhead, endive, green leaf, iceberg, red leaf, romaine

Mushrooms

Peppers (green, red)

Pickles (Bubbie's only)

Sauerkraut (Bubbie's or other brand with live probiotic only. Bubbie's is best because each batch is different, so you get a variety of balance in the probiotics.)

Scallions

Tomatoes

Watercress

Fruits

Local, in-season fruits

Avocado

Cantaloupe, oranges or
  tangerines

Coconut (fresh or
  unsweetened, shredded)

Lemon

Olives (high salt, so in
  moderation)

Peach

Pear

Plum

Raspberries, strawberries,
  blackberries

Watermelon

Apples are on the maybe, maybe-not list. They can cause bloating and gas. On the flip side, they can also help regulate your bowels, so pay attention to how your body responds.

Dried fruits aren't recommended because not only do most have a lot of added sugar, they can also cause stomach issues. They are also dehydrated, so if you eat them, you'll need extra water intake.

Carbohydrates

(starchy)

Beans (cooked only)

Edamame

Hummus (made from garbanzo
  beans)

Lentils (cooked only)

Peas

Parsnips (a high-carb vegetable)

Plantains

Sweet potatoes or yams

Carbohydrate pseudograins

(If you are sensitive to grains, this is your go-to list. Pay attention to how your body reacts. Professional opinions vary on this, so this list is based on least reactive to the body.)

Amaranth

Buckwheat (look for the hot cereal or pasta)

Millet (available in cereal and bread)

Quinoa (the pasta usually is made with corn, so best to use it on its own)

Teff

Wild rice (healthiest choice)

Carbohydrate grains

(organic only, limited amount)

Brown rice

Corn (organic only, in moderation and fresh, best to avoid while you are still restoring your health)

Einkorn

Rye

Slow-cooked oats

Sprouted grain bread

Whole wheat

Nuts

(These can be irritating or scrapy to a sensitive system, so pay attention to your response. They may need to be avoided in the early part of your health restoration process.)

Almonds (raw)

Cashews

Hazelnuts

Macadamia nuts

Pecans

Pine nuts

Pistachio

Seeds: chia, flax, hemp, pumpkin, sunflower, sesame

(Peanuts frequently are a bit moldy and can irritate the body. If you choose to eat peanuts or peanut butter, make sure that the ingredients are only peanuts and salt, no sugars.)

Dairy

(raw, organic, pasture-raised is best)

Blue cheese (unless you have a mold sensitivity)

Butter

Cheddar

Cottage cheese

Feta cheese

Goat

Heavy cream

Mozzarella

Parmesan cheese

Ricotta cheese

Swiss cheese

Whole milk (goat or cow)

Yogurt (plain, unsweetened, minimum fat at 2 percent)

Protein

(If you get game or other local meats with flavoring, such as sausage, be sure to check the ingredients yourself. Some people have significant flare-ups from local, healthy sourced meats that have chemicals added for flavor. If you ask the vendor if it's healthy, they may think it is. But they don't know as much as you do, so they may be incorrect. Be sure to check it yourself. All fish should be wild caught. All meats should be organic and grass-fed. All eggs should be organic, free-range, and grass-fed.)

Beef

Buffalo

Chicken

Cod

Eggs

Flounder

Game

Goat

Haddock

Halibut

Herring

Lamb

Sardines

Shellfish (lobster, shrimp, crab in limited amounts)

Tilapia

Tuna (limited amounts)

Turkey

Whitefish

A Note about Longevity and Vitality and Food: Today we are increasing the lifespan of people, but most people are not getting healthier as they live longer. They are on more and more medications and experiencing more and more disabilities.

If you've witnessed a loved one kept alive with medications and devices, you may be aware of suffering that you personally want to avoid. This isn't a natural process. It may be normal today—but it certainly isn't natural. And it is expensive.

In addition, the number one reason for bankruptcy in the US is medical bills. Women statistically experience more poverty than men as they get older. What I've seen in my patient population is women care for their husbands, spend quite a bit of their savings on their husband's care, outlive them, and end up in poverty.

What can you do to interrupt this cycle? And how can you enjoy a life of longevity without committing to a life of rabbit food?

If you consider people who have lived quality lives into their nineties and beyond, they often stick to native diets. As you look at native diets, you see real foods. One of the foods that used to be a staple is bread. Today, we have learned that wheat is bad for you and leads to gluten allergies and subsequent health problems. Many attribute this to the genetic modification of wheat.

But there is another difference.

The introduction of active dry yeast in the 1940s meant that you could make bread fairly quickly and didn't have to wait eight to ten hours for the bread to rise. That shortcut interrupted a long fermentation process that creates health for the human body.

When the fermentation process takes as long as it does with real sourdough bread, you get lactic acid, which supports gut bacteria. You also get the unleashing of numerous nutrients, which are lacking in modern bread.

Because so many habits and desires are ingrained in our DNA and passed from parent to child, is it any wonder that you may crave bread? You might even say that your craving for bread is in your DNA.

Basic sourdough has three ingredients: sea salt, water, and wheat. If you toss in the secret ingredient of love, now backed by science, you may be able to enjoy this treat again. Being healthy and enjoying a long life includes enjoying your food.

6

Poisons to Stop Putting In and On Your Body

Foods contain a gradient of health. A lot of foods out there aren't healthy for you, even though you are told they are.

In the last chapter I pointed out that the healthiest foods are the ones closest to the original state of the food when it is harvested. Getting rid of sugar, adding in more vegetables, possibly lowering your carbs, and getting off the mainstream junk food list—like candy bars and packaged treats—will obviously improve your health.

Such a practice will improve your health, but we are going to maximize your health.

The most often overlooked problem by the mainstream version of health is the chemicals in your food. Chemicals put a lot of stress on your body and do a slow chipping away at your health. Diet soda is probably one of the worst drinks available. There are alternatives, so you can wean yourself off (and avoid withdrawal symptoms).

The worst thing about diet soda is its link to Alzheimer's disease and dementia over the long term. The sweeteners mess with your nervous system, most often affecting the brain and cognition, but they can cause other neurological problems as well. And, of course, if you look at the ingredients of soda, they are loaded with chemicals, which are discussed in the interferences chapter.

Since much of this information about food risk is now being censored, you may need to look it up in alternative search engines.

If a food is in a package and has been premade, it is probably not healthy. There is a way to figure out how messed up it will make you: Pick up a packaged item from your pantry. Turn it over and look for the *Ingredients List*. Words that you don't understand indicate that they are probably chemicals.

Obviously, if you've studied chemistry, this might not work for you. But if you are a chemist, just imagine that you're not and try it. The more of these unknown words there are, the worse the food item is for you.

If you pick up something packaged and it has fewer than four or five ingredients, it is probably okay for you to eat. The fewer ingredients, the better. An exception to this is something like sprouted grain bread where the ingredients include a few different types of sprouted grains. Sprouted grains are fine for many people.

The food industry is full of marketing, so anything packaged with a label indicating that it is healthy for you may not be healthy for you.

Gluten-free foods are often full of chemicals and additives, including sugar. Chemicals are bad for you. If there are chemicals in your food, they are poisoning you and are, therefore, unhealthy.

Chemicals are used in the farming process in many parts of the world. These are poison and unhealthy. There are often legal cases about them. (Think Erin Brockovich.)

The Poison Game

This is a game to play when shopping. I made this up in the grocery store when I started healing myself and was overwhelmed with the amount of thinking I was putting into every little thing I was purchasing, and I was in a desperate situation with my health.

To keep shopping simple and fast, I sometimes play The Poison Game. Yes, calling it poison is dramatic. But if you're sick enough, it's also true.

The Poison Game Rules: Go into the store. Look around. Label foods as poison or not poison.

Baseline: If it's poison, you can't get it. If it's not poison, you can buy and eat it.

Gradient: If it's been labeled poison, but there is no other choice, choose the one that is *least poison*. You have won the game when you leave the store, and all food items in your cart are *not poison* or *least poison*.

If you are very sick and on the fast track to recovery, then you only win if all items are *not poison*.

Example 1: I enter the grocery store. My goal is all organic or sustainably raised. I'm in the vegetable section. I walk by the avocados—poison? Poison because they were probably sprayed. But they aren't on the EWG's annual dirty dozen list (www.EWG. org). So they are *least poison*. I put them in my cart.

Regular tomatoes—poison; organic tomatoes—not poison. I head to the organic section. Not poison. I get my zucchini. The cucumbers are squishy. Is this something required for a recipe for an event such as Thanksgiving dinner? No. What else can I get for a vegetable? Carrots. Organic carrots. Not poison.

Moving on to the meat section. Lots of regular meat—poison. Organic meat—not poison. (Typically, if you are on a budget and need meat, the regular meat would be *least poison* because the other option would be canned meat. Currently, the price for regular meat matches local and grass-fed meat.)

Since I get local meat where they are grazing on land that isn't sprayed—that is my personal *not poison*—but in the grocery store, this is the best I can get.

I walk to the back of the store and head to the frozen section. To my left are all the aisles in the middle of the store. Poison, poison, poison.

I get to the freezer section. Poison everywhere. I head to the fruit section. Poison next to not poison.

I'm on a budget, so I can opt for those as *least poison* where I can. Pineapple is peeled, so that is *least poison*. The regular blueberries are sprayed with stuff, so they are poison, and I get the organic of those.

I walk through the store by the bakery. Poison, poison, poison. I notice the freshly baked bread smell. Poison.

Example 2: I needed to get cauliflower for cauliflower mashed potatoes for Thanksgiving. The organic fresh ones were moldy looking, and the other ones would get moldy by the time I could get to make it and before I would get back to the store.

I went to the frozen section. They were out of organic (not poison). The nonorganic foods were flavored (poison). I had to look around to find the riced cauliflower that was without flavors (least poison).

That was a win and counted in my cart. If I had been in the beginning phases, I would've done a pass on the cauliflower. If you are starting your healing journey and your health is in a delicate condition or easily unbalanced, it is best to stick with the straight-up *not poison*.

Do your best. Progress. Not perfection.

Here is the gradient of healthy foods I discussed from best to worst:

Best

Local,* organic or sustainably raised, fresh

Local,* regular farming, fresh

Nonlocal, organic, fresh

Nonlocal, organic, frozen

Nonlocal, regular farming

Nonlocal, regular farming, frozen

Organic, canned

Regular farming, canned

Worst

*Local is going to have the best nutrients for you based on your location and are often most easily found at your local farmers' market. It will also be the freshest. You are a part of your environment—the air you breathe, the water you drink. So having local food contributes to your health.

Nonlocal won't be as fresh, and it won't have the nutrients you need based on where you live.

Canned foods are dead and will leech some chemicals. They are still far, far better than a candy bar or other more processed foods.

Sugar and Sweeteners: As you start reading the ingredients on packaged and processed foods, you'll notice that sugar is in just about everything. Sugar itself isn't bad, but because it is in everything, it is creating inflammation in your body, and you likely have some level of addiction to it.

It's not your fault. It's just how the system is set up.

Sugar is addictive. Not only that, but it messes with your organ health and creates cravings. When you eat, your body is looking for fuel in the form of nutrients. Foods with added sugar and low in nutrients (packaged meals included) make it far too easy to continue eating without ever getting full.

The lower the nutrients and the higher the sugars, the easier it is to keep eating without being satisfied. This happens because your body is seeking nutrients in the food that it isn't getting. So this lack of nutrients causes you to keep eating. And eating. And eating.

It is almost as if this mix forces you to keep going and forces you into gluttony.

The best way to stop this cycle is to increase the fats in your diet, and increase the nutritional foundation of what you are eating.

With no off-switch to the way most foods are made, gluttony has become the norm. Again, it's not your fault. It's just how things are right now.

Fortunately, once you discover just how good you feel without sugar, it becomes easier to make the choice and figure out how to graciously say "no thank you" when it is offered.

Going overboard on the other side (overly restricted) is unlikely. But to keep things balanced, consider biblical feast days. No matter which calendar you look at, there are fewer feast days than regular. My favorite version has feast days about twice a month, except in January. January is cold and a time when eating a lot can be healthful. At least in the northern hemisphere.

If you use that as a guide, you will eat moderately most of the month, then have some fun with your food a couple of days a month. This gives you something to look forward to and also ensures that you are eating for energy and not for gluttony.

If you have a spiritual text that you use, you might check it for guidance as well.

So what do you do for your treats if you aren't using sugar? It may be hard to believe right now, but fruit begins tasting sweeter, and if you are eating organic, you'll notice that it tastes so much sweeter and is more flavorful than the others.

Natural sugar substitutes are also an option. Anything in a yellow, blue, or pink packet is a toxin to your body and needs to be avoided. Corn syrup is to be avoided because most corn in the United States is heavy with toxins.

Sugar alcohols end with the letters -*ol*. This is easy to remember because alco*hol* also ends with the letters -*ol*. Alcohol stresses the liver, but so does sugar alcohol. It has been linked to chronic liver cancer and liver cancer. Erythritol has been shown to prevent cavities and is found in chewing gum, sodas, and other foods. It is still an alcohol sugar.

The health food stores have many items with erythritol in them because it is a trend and considered a better option. If you are sticking with level 2 health, then it certainly is the best choice for you.

This brings us to another point. Just because an item is in a health food store doesn't mean that it is truly healthy. Many items have sugar. Organic sugar is still sugar. Erythritol is still an alcohol sugar.

As you explore your local health food store or the health food section in your local grocery store, you may notice that most of these foods are level 2 or higher. So if your quest is for level 3, you'll have to think about what you are purchasing. This is especially true about processed, packaged, and premade foods.

If you are a soda drinker, you might be wondering what to drink. The mainstream wisdom is that diet soda is better for you than regular. This is level 1 thinking. Diet sweeteners and sugar are both poisons to the body. The soda from the United States is made with corn syrup. If you are able to get sodas from Mexico, those are made with cane sugar and are the best option of the three (non-optimal/bad) options.

To be clear, none of these is an option for a healthy body, so don't take it as a stamp of approval for drinking soda. It's not.

There are sodas with a hint of flavor that will give you the bubbly experience and a touch of flavor. But don't worry, as you get off the chemicals and your body becomes healthier, the strong chemical flavor of sodas will become apparent, and sodas will begin to lose their appeal.

Sugar substitutes to consider include monkfruit and stevia. These are the two best options. But buyer beware! Those are usually blended with erythritol. (Tip: To know if a sweetener is an alcohol sugar, just look at the end of the word. Alcohol ends with -ol, as does erythritol.)

Coconut palm sugar is widely available. It is better for you than the fake sugars and regular sugar. In the debate about it, some alternative practitioners say it is as bad as sugar. I disagree. It also can easily be used as a replacement for regular sugar in your favorite recipes at a 1:1 ratio.

Local raw honey and maple syrup have higher sugar content, but they are about as close to the source as you can get with natural sweeteners. If you have begun cutting out processed foods, then you are getting less sugar overall and this becomes less of a concern.

Short list of foods to avoid:

- Soda, especially diet soda

- Packaged foods with more than four ingredients or packaged food with chemicals

- Sugar and things that turn into sugar

Short list of foods to eat:

- Fresh, real food.

If your food, without the interference of processing or outright laboratory creation, had a mother, swam in water, walked on land, was pulled or harvested directly from the soil or was plucked from a tree, then it is considered fresh, real food.

Poisons in Things We Put On Our Bodies

This is basic. There are ingredients in our self-care and home care products that are full of chemicals and metals. You are, quite literally, surrounded. The more you have in your physical environment, the more stress it puts on your body.

Individually and in limited amounts, they are considered harmless. But there is an abundance of chemicals, and they are in everything.

Years ago I saw a study from the 1980s saying that there were over 30,000 chemicals in our food, water, and air that we were exposed to weekly. I can no longer find the study, but, logically, there are more toxins today than there were in the 1980s. The University of California is doing plenty of research regarding the toxins in our environment today.

And there are, quite frankly, far too many to cover in this book. You can research many products with the Environmental Working Group. If you have a favorite product, hold off until you've gone through the rest of them.

Basically, you start with the least toxic you can find for a product that you don't have an attachment to. Since toxins interfere with your health, they are referred to as *interferences* and are covered in the next chapter.

7

Interferences to (a.k.a. Destroyers of) Your Body's Health

Your body's foundation of true health is achieved by having the right quality and quantity of food, movement, thoughts, and feelings. The healthier your body is in these areas, the less welcoming it will be to the *interferences*. However, interferences do get in because our world is inundated with them. The healthier you are, the faster the supplementation works to get your body balanced again.

Let's talk about the interferences.

Viruses and Bacteria

These cause both mild and severe illnesses, the flu, colds, bugs in the stomach or colon, the cause of diarrhea, and more.

We have had many patients who have been positive for COVID. It's an ugly illness. Everyone who got on a supplement program targeted at strengthening the body to fight off COVID has gotten better. Remember, supplements don't heal anything. They make your body stronger. Nutritional protocols are developed to get results. And they do.

Quickest Way to Stop a Cold Before It Settles In

Health tip: If you feel as if you may be catching something, then putting 3 percent hydrogen peroxide in each ear helps knock it out. If it bubbles, it's knocking out bacteria or virus. You have to do this before the interference becomes a full-blown illness. Start noticing your signs, and you can nip them in the bud. Some signs include sneezing a couple of times, itchy ears, or a tickle in the throat.

If you do the peroxide because you feel as if you're fighting something off, but it doesn't bubble, the main interference you are fighting off is not bacteria or virus but metals or chemicals instead. In this case, taking the correct supplement for chemical and metal detoxification will reduce or eliminate your symptoms.

Metals and Chemicals

Various metals and chemicals are found in your self-care products, cleaning products, food, water, and air. Their number is increasing. These are not good for you. Period.

There are so many of them that it would take hours to go through and cross-reference them with any symptoms you might be having. As mentioned in another chapter, the Environmental Working Group has done all the work for you. You can put products into a search database on their website and find out about your favorite products.

Symptoms of having metal or chemical toxicity often mimic symptoms of coming down with something on the superficial level. At a deeper level, metals and chemicals are connected to just about any health issue you may be facing.

One of the most interesting observations I've had over the years regarding metals and chemicals is that detoxification followed by uterine nutritional support has reduced or more often eliminated menstrual cramps in my female patients who also experienced fewer miscarriages and increased fertility. We have also seen surprise pregnancies, as well as planned ones.

Parasites

Parasites are not as exciting as movies would have you believe. We all have parasites in our bodies; we just want to make sure that the ones we are hosting are good for us.

Yes, parasites sounds disgusting. Nobody wants to think about it. I won't delve into it too far here. However, they are quite common. Kids and pets are the biggest culprits for bringing them into the home. They get in through food and your nose, mouth, and skin.

Feeling like something is crawling under your skin is a symptom of parasites. As is sugar addiction. Parasites somehow take over your body and force you to eat (binge on) sugar.

It's often best to work with a practitioner for parasites because the parasite detoxification process can be complicated. A lot of popular detoxification programs can cause serious damage to the body. If you choose to do it on your own, be careful.

Fungus and Mold

These are found in nature and are prevalent in humid areas. They thrive in moist environments.

Fungus and mold frequently are found in people who have metals, parasites, or both. They can also be present if the stomach and intestinal bacteria have been compromised from years of unhealthy eating and numerous rounds of antibiotics.

Scars

Scars are treated to soften them up and improve the nerve flow that has been interfered with. Scars are treated with an oil.

There have been interesting stories about scars such as these:

- A decrease in a seemingly unrelated symptom when treating the scar. A finger scar affecting digestion, a leg scar affecting a headache.

- Something coming out of the body, such as a piece of metal or fiber. It will create a pimple and then come out.

- The softening of the thick birthing scars at the perineum.

Detoxing

Detoxing is the process of getting the toxins out of the body. It starts with opening the *exit channels* by making some diet and lifestyle changes suggested in the next section. An exit channel is the channel or pathway of exit for the toxins:

- Sweat through the skin (including eyes)

- Breath through the lungs

- Urine through the kidneys and bladder

- Feces through the colon

To think that your body can just detoxify without added assistance through strategic dietary support and nutritional supplementation is optimistic and ignores the fact that there is massive pollution in our world.

Every time you drink unfiltered water from the tap, or eat any kind of processed food or eat fresh foods that were sprayed with chemicals, you are putting more toxins into your body that your body has to deal with.

The detoxification support supplements help the body go through the process of cleaning out. In the old days, we didn't need supplements because our food source was of a much higher quality with more nutrients and fewer pollutants. We also know more about health now.

One effective way to get the process of detoxification started is with a detox footbath. This opens the exit channels. There is a whole science to it that is too much for this book. But what I can tell you is that patients who use it need fewer detox supplements when they do the footbath.

When I introduced it into my practice, every patient that did the footbaths dropped down on their detoxification supplements. If you want to get one, get a quality supplement. It is true that you get what you pay for

Other than that, there are many supplements to help get toxins out. Check with your natural health provider and check out www.ToxinsInMyLife.com.

The reason to have professional support for detoxing is because of the possibility of a detox reaction, which has some people thinking that it's dangerous. Professionals who don't recommend detoxification are likely not educated in either the benefits or the process. Those who believe a severe reaction is just part of the process haven't been introduced to alternatives.

A detox reaction occurs when the interferences are leaving your body at a rate that is greater than what your body can handle. Your body isn't strong enough or ready for the dump of toxins that is occurring. By having an individualized detox support protocol, you can avoid the reaction but still get the benefits.

If detoxification has been intense, it can take weeks and months to recover. Detoxification is necessary, but it can also be done in a more kind, gentle, and loving way by using strategic nutritional supplementation to build up the body's ability to remove the toxins, strengthen the body, and then slowly let the toxins out in a way that is nurturing to the body. This works best with muscle testing so the various nuances of support can be monitored and adjusted.

By working with a professional who looks at the detoxification from this perspective, you can have the exit process monitored so that you have little to no symptoms. There are rarely symptoms when the process is monitored correctly. At most, the symptoms will be minor, such as a slight rash, a bout of diarrhea that goes away quickly, bad breath, or smelly bowels.

When you support your body throughout the detoxification process, your body has more energy to focus on your health and vitality.

Here are some common examples of metal and chemical interferences:

- Aluminum is in tin foil and antiperspirants. It is linked to dementia and Alzheimer's.

- Fluoride is in toothpaste and city water. Fluoride calcifies around your pineal gland, which is the part of your body that helps you create and connect to God/the Divine/Source.

- Glyphosate is used in farming. It is linked to cancer. It is still widely used and sold in the United States but banned in many other countries.

- Food dyes are sometimes made from bugs and other gross ingredients. They have been linked to cancer.

- Chemical cleaners are linked to asthma and other health issues.

Some common symptoms of toxicity are these:

- You can't walk down the scented aisles at the grocery store without a headache, sneezing, or feeling nauseous.

- You get a little sick after you eat, but you're not sure how or what it is connected to. You can't figure it out.

- You can't drink water because it makes you sick.

- Your skin itches a lot.

- You have frequent headaches.

- You are tired and you can't get un-tired no matter how much you rest or sleep.

- Your brain is fuzzy and/or you feel as if you are always in a fog.

- You are frequently nauseous when you are exposed to certain scents.

- You have seasonal allergies.

What You Can Do about Interferences Right Now

Exercise, eat natural foods, and start moving your thoughts and conversations away from fixating on worry, stress, and oppression, and moving them toward problem-solving, gratitude, and appreciation.

What you can do now to start opening your exit channels:

Drink water: Drinking water is essential. Your body is made up of mostly water. If water bothers your stomach, it could mean the acid balance is off in your stomach and/or there are insufficient digestive enzymes in your system.

There may be chemicals in your water that are irritating your stomach. A water filter is helpful. If you can't afford one, the water from your faucet is better than sodas.

Drinking 1 ounce of water per pound of body weight is the minimum to give you the best results. Working up to a gallon a day will give your body plenty of health benefits.

Your skin: Your biggest organ is your skin. Whatever goes on your skin, goes in you. Natural lotions are best.

Lotions can be expensive, so look for locally made options. Coconut oil works well for many people and is budget-friendly. Watching what is in your skincare and your makeup is important, but unless you have skin problems, you can put this low on your list.

Drinking the gallon of water also helps flush out your skin and you'll notice it becomes clearer and younger looking. Skin is one of the detoxification channels in your body. If you are prone to skin issues, it is usually your body detoxing.

Your lungs: What you breathe in can make you sick. Nature is often blamed when chemicals are the problem.

In farm country, seasonal allergies are often most helped with a detox protocol for chemicals. Exercising enough to where you breathe heavily helps your body remove toxins. Try yoga, running, or fast walking.

Your stomach: Anything you eat and drink should be as pure and as close to nature as possible. Green leafy vegetables help your body remove toxins. Eating four cups a day of fresh vegetables is a great rule of thumb. As long as the vegetables aren't doused in oil, this amount supports weight loss and the reduction of acid reflux.

8

Maximizing What You Put In Your Body

To maximize what you put into your body, you will need to supplement the foods you eat. People in excellent health prioritize taking supplements. People in level 4 definitely take supplements.

But all supplements are not made the same. Supplement claims are not regulated by the government. The supplements you get at the regular store may or may not contain what they claim on the label. The professional brands used by natural health doctors do. They are held to account by the natural doctors, who are far more exacting with the manufacturers and have higher standards than the government.

Different Types of Supplements

There are three different types of supplements: synthetic nutritional supplements, natural nutritional supplements, and whole food supplements.

Synthetic nutritional supplements and natural nutritional supplements are both called, simply, nutritional supplements, which are combinations of dietary ingredients such as vitamins, minerals, amino acids, and enzymes.

The body has to work hard to get the synthetic nutritional supplements to work in the body. Unfortunately, this describes the majority of over-the-counter supplements.

Natural supplements are sourced from foods. In a body that is trying to strengthen and recover from disease and illness, this is an excellent option for strengthening the organs in the body. These are used by many functional medicine doctors and natural health doctors and practitioners.

Whole food supplements are condensed foods and are the best way to move a body into a state of level 4 health. Because your body is given the whole food, doses tend to be higher, but long-term results are also better.

The nutrients in our foods have declined steadily over the past few decades due to modern farming practices. The soil doesn't have the nutrients necessary for plants, so nutrients have to be added to the soil. The nutrients added aren't the full spectrum of what is healthy, but enough to help the plants grow.

Even in the 1960s, there was a noticeable decline in the nutrients in food. The situation is even worse today. When you provide your body with the right quality and quantity of food, it will be healthy. With the decrease of nutrients in foods, you would have to eat far more than is reasonable to get the nutrients your body needs to operate at level 3 or 4. Whole food supplements are the best way to increase the quality of food without increasing the quantity.

Since nutrients from food are what feed your organs, it only makes sense to take condensed whole foods to keep your organs at their best.

Don't Make This Mistake When Getting Your Health Back

Restoring your health means that your organs can do their job through the whole food nutrients you provide it. Whole food supplements support the restoration of your organs in their natural ability to function, including their ability to detoxify your body.

Most people use symptom-based reasoning for taking supplements. You take them until the symptom goes away. Then you stop taking them. This is a big mistake with health restoration. Your symptoms will go away long before the organ has been restored. It takes one to three years to restore an organ. Once it is restored, it still needs nutrients.

A pattern I see with those who use symptom-based reasoning is this: You have an organ that isn't working. Let's use the heart as an example. You feed it correctly with whole food supplements. You change your diet and your environment. Your heart starts working better. Your medical doctor gives you routine tests to check the progression of your condition. Your doctor takes you off your blood pressure medications. You feel great. You believe you have fixed your heart. You stop feeding it correctly. You stop taking your supplements and start eating how you used to. Your blood pressure goes back up. So you get back on your medication.

Next is an example of someone who understands the importance of feeding their organs: You have an organ that isn't working. I will continue with the heart as an example. You feed it correctly with whole food supplements. It starts working. You feel great. You believe you have fixed your heart. You continue taking your supplements. You are able to exercise more and be more active. Your supplements for your heart reduce over the next year. Your medical doctor takes you off your blood pressure medications.

You are ready to feed your next organ. You start working on your thyroid. You are eating foods recommended for your thyroid condition. You continue taking the right supplements for your heart. You add the right supplements to feed your thyroid. Your prescribing medical doctor starts helping you reduce your medications.

Next, you decide to tackle your antidepressants. You are confident and excited because you are getting healthier every year. You feel amazing. When your organs begin functioning well, you won't have symptoms. This doesn't mean that you should take the nutrients away that are feeding them.

Symptom-based thinking is consistent with level 1 and level 2 thinking. This isn't true when we are talking about maximizing organ function. The way we can tell if the organ is starting to function with your food and some simple supplements is through blood tests or muscle testing. The muscle testing is used to determine how long is long enough to stay on them.

A common occurrence has happened recently with the COVID vaccine and boosters. Vaccines have additives in them that need to be detoxified by the body for optimal functioning. This is true of all modern vaccines. The vaccine will create an immune response in the body. A bulk of the toxins will leave the body, but there is enough left in the system to create problems for people with more sensitive bodies, like those with the MTHFR gene mutation. The detoxification gets these remnants out. It does not affect the immune response. That process has already been put into motion.

Vaccines and Detoxification

You can think of the vaccine as a diesel truck in an enclosed building. The truck is the vaccine. The small, enclosed building is your body. You are standing in the building, and you represent an organ. Let's say the heart.

The vaccine starts the truck and the truck leaves to do its work. The truck leaves behind fumes or toxins. If you stay inside, you might not feel good or start coughing. But if you open the windows and let the fumes out, it won't affect you as much.

The immune response is the truck leaving the building. That process has happened. The detoxification process is opening the windows.

Practitioners use many protocols for supporting their patients who get vaccines. With my protocol, patients start the protocol the day of the shot, and it usually takes a month for the process to complete.

When the COVID vaccine came out, my patients started with the typical protocol. But patients were coming in after the month with heart palpitations, anxiety, and depression. With the muscle testing, I was able to find that they had to do triple the detoxification for the COVID vaccine. This was new.

Once they started back on the detoxification supplements, the palpitations, anxiety, and depression reduced and went away. There was a pattern of extra support needed for family genetic conditions, heart support, and nervous system support.

By getting my patients on the detoxification protocol and providing the extra nutritional support, these symptoms went away. Their bodies were able to adapt and become strong again.

It can take one to three years to restore your body to a maintenance level. Any stress put in or on your body increases the amount of time it takes to restore. The longer you have had a condition and the more severe it is, the longer it takes.

Most people, if they stop taking their supplements when their body still wants them, will not feel the symptoms come back right away. It could take weeks or years, but it will likely happen because the body will start adapting again.

The whole food supplements are strengthening the function of the organs such that they begin to thrive again and there is no longer an environment for disease or illness. When you stop giving your body the nutrients it needs, that foundational support has been removed. The organ is once again left to its own devices. And the body will adapt as long as it can.

If health at level 1 or level 2 is your goal, then getting off the supplements is likely appropriate for you.

If you want to be at level 3 or level 4, then continuing to take the supplements is your best option. It may be obvious to you that those at levels 3 and 4 are most successfully fighting the natural aging process.

As you work on restoring your health and become better able to understand how your body works, the mystery of why things are happening starts to go away. You are able to self-assess and make corrections. The peace of mind is remarkable.

Here is a brief outline of what you can do to improve your health starting now.

Pick one activity and do it for a couple of weeks, then add another one. They are in no particular order, so pick whatever works for you to start with.

1. Change diet (no supplements necessary).

2. Control interferences (no supplements necessary—you are getting items out of your home and environment that cause harm, perhaps using EWG as a resource).

3. Support then restore digestive function (supplements helpful): You can't absorb nutrients if your digestive system isn't working. Supplements help any or all of the digestive organs, including parotid glands (saliva), esophagus, stomach, liver, pancreas, gallbladder, small intestines, and large intestines.

4. Remove interferences, a.k.a. detoxification: Toxins leave through your skin, eyes, bowels, urine, and breath. These are supported with supplements. If you detox too fast, you may get symptoms, like bad breath or pimples. If you have these already, your body is trying to detox. This is accomplished by including green vegetables, exercise, and supplements.

5. Restore organ function: Take supplements to fuel the organs; eat organ meats, real foods, do moderate exercise, practice meditation/prayer with gratitude and love. In this phase, it is time to talk to your medical doctor about getting off other medications.

6. Maintain and maximize organ function: Take supplements to continue fueling the organs by fine-tuning all elements of #5 including real foods, exercise, meditation/prayer with gratitude and love.

If you have had to restore an organ to get off medication, it is realistic to assume that you will be giving targeted nutrition to that organ for up to three years or more. Examples: kidney disease, pancreas for diabetes, liver from alcohol abuse, heart from heart disease, joints, and muscles from overuse.

Nutrients to Target Organs

Health tip: If you have an organ that's failing, such as your heart, eat that organ. You can get these online or at your farmers' market. If you don't want to eat it, then find it within a whole food supplement.

One of the most nutrient-dense organs is the liver. Because it is a detoxification organ, it is also very clean.

If you want my list of recommended whole food supplements that support detoxification and organ restoration, you can get it at www.WholeFoodSupplementList.com. Since there are knock-offs of many supplements, some made in other countries, it's safest to get them directly from a doctor who carries them.

Any time you put interferences in your environment or body, your body will respond and will need support. If you are on medications or struggling to overcome a disease, it's best to work with a professional who is trained in helping people restore their health.

If you have tried everything on your own, have a stack of supplements in your cupboard or around your house, and you haven't gotten the results you are looking for, then it's time to reach out to a professional, and I address how to find the right professional in the final chapter of this book.

For most people, this is a journey. You will have doctors that help you to a point, and then it is time to move on. But before we explore what to look for in a professional, let's look at the last two things you can control: movement and your environment—internal and external.

9

The Truth about 10,000 Steps

"I did my 10,000 steps!"

The measure of 10,000 steps is a great start on your journey to health, especially if you have not been moving. If those early steps are difficult for you, then 10,000 steps is a worthwhile goal from which you can launch your improved health. However, if you want health and vitality—movement is part of the puzzle. Having 10,000 steps as your end goal will not get you there.

The person who does 10,000 steps will be healthier than the person who walks 2,000 steps. The person who eats perfectly and takes all the right supplements and doesn't do more than 10,000 steps is going to be healthier than someone who does all the exercise but doesn't manage the chemistry of their body with nutrients.

The person who combines quality, regular exercise with the right foods and supplements is going to be healthier than either of those. And the person who combines the right exercise, food, and environment is going to be the healthiest of all.

Remember, foods fuel your body. If you are eating foods that create inflammation, it is harder to move. If you are eating foods that give energy to your body, it is easier to move.

The right amount of exercise is critical to achieve level 3 and 4 health.

As with everything, the following recommendations for exercise are to be individualized. If you use a wheelchair, you still need to move. If you are bedridden and paralyzed, can you exercise your hand? It is important that you start with where you are.

If your body isn't working well for you, your greatest challenge may be overcoming the unkind messages and frustration that you are directing toward your body. Shifting those to love and appreciation will make a world of difference for you.

When a body is limited by inflammation and pain, improving your body's chemistry with detoxification and nutrients will help. Your body is made to move. Your job as the custodian of your body is to make sure that you can keep moving.

It is no secret that a sedentary lifestyle contributes to the diseases that we see today. Movement of the right amount and quality will keep you healthy. Not enough and too much exercise is not the right mix.

But what is enough exercise?

We can go to the World Health Organization to find out what exercise is recommended for those living at the top of the paradigm of level 1 health and possibly level 2. The experts at WHO say you "should do at least 150–300 minutes of moderate-intensity aerobic physical activity" (about 20-45 minutes a day); "or at least 75-150 minutes of vigorous-intensity aerobic physical activity; or an equivalent combination of moderate- and vigorous-intensity activity throughout the week" (about 11–20 minutes a day). And they say "adults should also do muscle-strengthening activities at a moderate or greater intensity that involve all major muscle groups on 2 or more days a week, as these provide additional health benefits."

If you want level 3 or level 4 health, then this is your starting point.

For the purpose of moving up the ladder to level 4 health, exercise can be distinguished by three groups: targeted, recovery, and walking.

Targeted exercise works the muscles of your cardiovascular system and your musculoskeletal system. The cardiovascular system is your heart muscle and your ability for endurance activities, like running or kayaking. The musculoskeletal system is your muscles and joints throughout your body. These are strengthening activities.

Exercise Recommendation for Level 4 Health

Targeted exercise should be 45 minutes minimum per day, 4 to 5 days a week minimum (6 is best)

- 3 days of exercise targeting increasing your heart rate, with the goal of your maximum target heart rate (below)

- 3 days of exercise targeting weights

- A mix of strengthening and cardiovascular on the same day to receive the benefit

Recovery exercise should be done at least once a week to stretch and treat your muscles and joints kindly for all their hard work. Lengthening and stretching the muscles will help prevent injury. Include foam rolling, mobilization, stretching, and the MELT method.

The MELT method is a self-treatment that rehydrates the connective, myo-fascial tissue throughout your body, reducing pain and increasing flexibility. If you have pushed your body over the last six days, your body will thank you. Skipping this type of exercise or mobilization will have your muscles tighten up and can lead to injury.

The target heart rate for cardiovascular exercise depends on your age and your health.

The following recommendation is directly from the American Heart Association. If you have heart issues, stay within the target heart rate zone of 50 to 85 percent. The higher you get on the list, the better. If your heart is damaged, stay in the lower end until you have restored its function and can safely work up to 85 percent.

Keep in mind that this chart comes from within the medical system. Those who have restored their health can safely get to a higher target heart rate for their age. However, don't get cocky and jump up to a higher range until the rest of your health is on point. And make sure to check with your trusted healthcare provider to determine if that rate is right for you.

When in doubt, go with the lower target heart rate. This is a marathon, not a sprint. Slow and steady wins the race. Being kind to yourself definitely helps you win the race.

Age	Target Heart Rate Zone (50 to 85 percent)
20 years	100–170 beats per minute (bpm)
30 years	95–162 bpm
35 years	93–157 bpm
40 years	90–153 bpm
45 years	88–149 bpm
50 years	85–145 bpm
55 years	83–140 bpm
60 years	80–136 bpm
65 years	78–132 bpm
70 years	75–128 bpm

Walking is a category of its own. It is best done daily, outside in fresh air. It is in addition to the targeted exercises.

You can walk with your spouse or partner, your kids, your friends, your dog, or alone. You can walk with intention, to clear your mind, create intentions, and allow your body to move freely. You can walk quickly or slowly.

We were meant to walk.

Walking with proper posture sets a strong foundation to prevent injuries. Walk straight and tall with your shoulders back and down and your stomach tucked in. Walk up hills to work on your glute muscles.

Walking improves your mental health and your physical health. Breathe in the fresh air and look around at your environment. Looking at the items around you and focusing on them is calming to your body and your mind. Walking outside is the perfect time to visualize the future you want to create. Get into the feeling of your future, healthy self.

Two walks a day are always an option. A slow, calming walk can be viewed as a recovery exercise or a brisk, intentional power walk can be a targeted exercise.

Managing Your Body for Movement

Just because the people around you are slowing down and getting less healthy doesn't mean you need to. However, having a body that moves well doesn't happen without managing it well. It is important to push yourself. But if you are prone to pushing yourself too hard, you will have injuries. If you push yourself too little, you will have minimal progress.

Overtraining is when you push yourself too hard and injure yourself. If you are prone to pushing yourself too hard, you will need to learn temperance regarding daily exercise to avoid injury. Undertraining limits your health improvement.

This is a balance that you will discover for yourself as you exercise more frequently.

For the sake of safety, pushing yourself too little is better for you than pushing yourself too hard. In either case, working with a professional trainer or joining a group class where you can get feedback from the instructor may be a good option for you.

Limitations in the movement of your musculoskeletal system are helped by a physical therapist at levels 1 and 2 or a chiropractor at levels 2, 3, and 4. A good physical therapist and a good chiropractor work at all levels. Having both is your best choice.

As you move up the health ladder and get to level 4, a chiropractor will keep your joint movement healthy and optimized, which will keep your muscles moving optimally and help prevent injury and improve function. The physical therapist will help your muscle movement and recovery.

Strengthening all your muscles puts beneficial stress on the nervous system, so it fuels your body's strength, power, and stamina. Power yoga, jogging, weightlifting, and cross-training are some options. Listen to your body.

Too Stressed to Exercise

The adrenal glands are the stress glands of the body. Many people today are suffering from adrenal fatigue or exhaustion. Symptoms of adrenal fatigue or exhaustion include having heart palpitations when walking or doing targeted exercises. In this case, start with soothing recovery exercises like gentle yoga or tai chi. Use light weights or no weights. Take slow walks with many pauses.

Do this as you feed your adrenal glands with the appropriate nutrients and herbs to help them recover. As your health improves, you will be able to gently increase your exercise capacity. You will learn what your limits are through trial and error. But never stop moving. That is key.

Exercise might be helping more than you realize. The nutrients in your body are delivered to your organs by your blood. Everything you ingest is brought throughout your body with blood. Your blood circulates better and with more oxygen when you exercise. Oxygen destroys diseases in your body. Increasing oxygen in your body improves your immune system.

And exercising is the simplest way to do this.

When you push yourself enough, you will get an endorphin rush, which lowers depression and anxiety while increasing a feeling of joy. This is called a runner's high when it occurs from running or jogging.

Exercising also increases your ability to enjoy and engage in activities that make life enjoyable—walking, hiking, lifting—it just makes life better.

Notice how you talk to yourself while exercising. Are you comparing yourself to others? Are you telling yourself that you are ugly? Fat? Too old? Saggy? That you're not good at it?

If you are, please stop. That is mean and unkind. Would you tolerate someone saying something like that to someone you love? It is also in the judgment category and is the energetic imprint of level 1. If you relate to yourself at level 1, you'll stay at level 1.

Here are some options for how to address your body at level 3 or 4 while exercising:

I'm so proud of you. You are doing an amazing job. That was hard and you did it! You finished doing it, even though you are tired. Good job. You are so beautiful/handsome. Look how well you are doing. You are amazing. I love you. I appreciate you. I love how hard you are working for me. You've got this. You worked so hard. Good for you.

If you are exercising at home, say these affirmations out loud. Words spoken out loud have more impact. It's up to you if you want to do it out loud at the gym.

My favorite expression to say to myself is, "Good job, Self!" Sometimes I accidentally say it out loud in public. When I do, I just figure someone around me needed to hear that. It's a simple and valid example of positive self-talk and gives others permission to do the same—something we need more of.

10

The Secret Behind the Environments that Make You Sick

Two environments you control can affect your health: the external and internal environments.

Internal Environment

The most impactful change you can make to your internal environment is how you talk to yourself and how you treat yourself. Many people have learned that they should speak positively to themselves, and they do it when they think about it. It is your automatic way of talking to yourself when you aren't consciously thinking about it where a big difference will be made.

Do you talk about parts of your body as if they are the enemy or out to get you? If you do this, you are reinforcing a neurological habit pattern that is creating more of what you are saying about them. That's level 1 behavior.

If your arm is giving you pain, it's crying out for help. Don't kick it when it's down. Would you do that to a kitten or puppy? Stop kicking it.

Your body has supported you despite all the junk you've put in it, the way you haven't exercised it, how you've talked to it, how you've pushed it beyond its limits. It's time to start showing your body some tenderness, care, and love.

When you look in the mirror, what do you say to yourself? If you notice that you're at the lower level, that is a success. Once you notice it, you can change your self-talk.

Sometimes people get frustrated when they notice how they are talking to themselves. Just remember that you have years of this thinking pattern ingrained in your neurological system. When you notice it, congratulate yourself on a job well done. Then, pick an alternative phrase for what feels loving and kind to yourself.

Any time you notice the damaging phrase, replace it with the loving one. The more you do this, the more it will become a habit. At some point, the damaging phrase will fall away and disappear.

External Environment

Whatever is in your external environment will affect your internal environment. The stronger your internal environment, the less of an effect the external will have.

Obviously, reducing the chemicals and metals as addressed in the interferences chapter is important. If they are in the air, they will enter through your lungs. If they are in the water, they enter your body through drinking or through your skin.

Do what you can to depollute your space.

On an energetic level, the external environment is what you are exposing your mind to. It can be tricky because, as you are uncovering the unsupportive external environments, you may discover that some external environments that you thought were supportive, aren't.

Is someone speaking to you with love and kindness? Or is the person speaking fear, disrespect, or hate? News sources and gossip, whether in person or on social media, are two areas where fear, disrespect, and hate are found.

Choosing your devotional or starting a meditation immediately shifts your environment to a higher level.

The more you keep your external and internal environments at a higher level, the closer you are to coming back in touch with the number one ingredient to truly getting healthy. That ingredient is your innate wisdom or gut instinct. When you are working with it and consistently taking its guidance, you know at a deep, confirming level when anything around you will be healthy or unhealthy for you.

Your Gut Instinct or Innate Wisdom

Your gut instinct is your own individual direct line to God, the Universe, the Divine, or whatever name you use. This is a gift that connects your physical body to the Divine wisdom that is a compass for your emotional health, physical health, and mental health.

We are all in touch with it on some level.

Your experience of that wisdom will become finely tuned toward your health as you continue down this path. The more you listen to it, the stronger and clearer the message becomes. Getting back in touch with your innate wisdom is the final piece that gives you access to maximizing your health and truly having health freedom.

Once you start making the connection between how good you feel with eating the right nutrients and exercising, you will understand on a deeper level that when you give your body what it needs, it naturally moves toward health.

Taking the correct, consistent action in a state of anger, hate, or fear will limit your progress and move you away from your innate wisdom. If you strive to have your heart full of love and appreciation while taking consistent action, you will get there.

The more you pay attention to that inner ticking of your innate wisdom, the more your life will organize in such a way that the right people and opportunities will appear in front of you.

However, often as you are starting out, it can be challenging to know if what you are listening to is innate wisdom or something else. Innate wisdom is always working in your favor.

Tools for Tapping into Your Innate Wisdom

If, like most people, you struggle with listening to your innate wisdom through all the noise that life throws at you, then learning how to muscle test and understanding its benefits and limitations could be a good option for you.

You can learn how to do this at home in my book *Intuition, Faith, and Freedom: The one at-home tool you need to avoid using medical intervention*. You just need someone to practice with. The book covers muscle testing as it relates to both religion and science. One chapter explains muscle testing with basic physics as well as quantum physics. Another chapter explores the question, "Is muscle testing biblical?"

If you struggle with being able to imagine a life of health and vitality, then my *Visualization to Manifestation* book will walk you through how to do this. Step by step.

If you are stuck in a mental or emotional pattern that you just can't shake with your prayer work or meditations, then working with EMBeR, Emotional & Mental Balancing & Repatterning, will help you.

EMBeR consists of TapOut–TapIn for shifting mental patterns and Emotional Imprint Identification and Release for releasing stuck emotional patterns linked to the different levels of health. TapOut is used to get the mental patterning that is negative out of your neurological framework. TapIn is used to insert statements that are loving and kind to you.

Muscle testing speeds up the process and progress with TapOut–TapIn because it is a direct, concrete line to your innate wisdom and is used to lessen the trial and error of working on patterns that are already handled by your subconscious so you can focus on the tasks that still need to be addressed.

You can use muscle testing to help determine exactly which phrases to use in a way that is safe and gentle.

These are all explained in detail in the muscle testing book. For deeper issues, it is best to work with a practitioner to help you navigate those murky, internal waters with love and compassion.

Part III

Working with a Professional

11

What Is Right for You?

Before determining whether working with a professional is right for you, start with identifying what health level you are in along with what your goal is. Be honest with yourself about whether or not you are willing to take action to move to a different level.

The majority of people will be comfortable in level 1. If this is the case for you, a traditional healthcare provider is best for you. If this is the level you are most satisfied with, then you are in good hands for your goals with the system as it is.

If you are at level 1 and want to get to level 2, many of the recommendations in this book will allow you to move into level 2. If you need help with some of the recommendations in the book, then something like our Nutrition Master Class might be best for you.

If you want to check your knowledge of what is healthy eating, you can take the free Nutrition Readiness Quiz at www.NutritionReadinessQuiz.com.

If, however, you want to start to experience the freedom and confidence that you are effectively fighting off the natural aging process while safely boosting your immune system, then a natural health professional will help get you into level 3 or 4. And even if you are currently at level 1, I've seen people get to level 3 in as little as two months. If it's possible for them, it's possible for you.

Self Quiz—Is Working with a Professional Right for You?

1. At what level of health are you now, and what level do you want to get to? 2? 3? 4? If there is a gap between the level where you are now and one of the higher levels, working with a professional may be right for you.

2. On a scale of 1 to 10 where 1 is no and 10 is willing to do whatever it takes, how willing are you to make changes in your life to restore your health? If you say 8, 9, or 10, you will have excellent results working with a professional. If it is a lower number, then working through this book on your own or starting with a functional blood test may be a good place to start.

3. If you want to get to level 3 or 4, how much are you willing or able to spend on your health? Health insurance does not pay for alternative health services. Health Share Accounts

often do. Determine what type of financial resources you are willing to allocate for improving your health and that of your family. Discuss this with your spouse or a partner and create a plan.

4. Do you have the support of people close to you for changing your lifestyle to be a healthier one? What changes can you agree on? Nothing interferes with health improvement more than an unsupportive family. On the flip side, nothing helps move your health forward like a supportive family member.

12

How to Choose
a Professional

Thousands of natural health practitioners are in practice outside of the medical system. Most natural health practitioners who deal with nutrition are adept at handling the interferences.

All of them can get you to level 2. Some will get you to level 3. And even fewer will get you to level 4, so do your homework, get references, and trust your gut.

For restoring and then enhancing your organs' function, you will want to find a practitioner who practices what they preach.

Not all practitioners will get you to maximal health. You'll want to work with someone who is at least a level ahead of you.

Consider your goals and where you want to get to. If they personally haven't gotten there, it is unlikely that they will get you there. If they have gotten there and fallen back due to life events, it is likely they can still get you there. They are merely human after all.

Here is a list of questions to ask before you move forward with a practitioner:

1. Has the practitioner gotten to at least where you want to in her own health? When she asks you what your goals are, then paint a picture for her. And ask her about her own health journey if she hasn't told you already.

2. Does she consider your entire history or just the past few years? Everything you have done and experienced in your life contributes to your health or dis-ease today. If she only looks at the past few years, she is missing some big pieces of the puzzle that is you.

3. Does her intake process for the main programs include a time for the practitioner to review your information before making recommendations? Or does she just jump in and start giving recommendations?

4. Does she accept everyone into care? Or does she refer out to other practitioners if she feels there is someone else who can help you better than she can?

5. Does she consider what you eat? What you eat is responsible for up to 70 percent of your health and healing.

6. Is it a program that is tailored to you? Or she recommending a cookie-cutter program that you are plugging yourself into? A cookie-cutter program is where everyone gets the exact same treatment protocol.

7. Is there a system that is used for analysis? A system means that she follows a set of procedures that allows for tracking patterns in your health. Any break in your pattern is an indication of a disruption of your health. For patients who have been following her recommended protocols, the cause of these pattern breaks can more easily be tracked when there is a system. Basically, you want her to use a standard system out of which an individualized program is created for you. To explain this, imagine being a bridesmaid. The style of the dress is the same for all the bridesmaids (system) but the measurements are individualized (program).

8. Is she willing to work with input from other practitioners? If you're trying to get to level 4, then have the level 4 practitioner as your main one, with input from others.

9. Does she use a method of assessment outside of those found in the regular medical paradigm, such as muscle testing or functional blood tests? Ideally, does she use both?

10. Does she have a program for supporting you in releasing emotional and mental imprints that are keeping you stuck? Or does she at least have someone to refer you to?

11. Does she address your digestive system, foundational support, and detoxification before giving you nutrients for other organs in your body?

12. Does she support you in getting off your medications safely by providing supplementation to support the organ in question while also using the recommendations from your prescribing doctor?

13. Is the office professional?

14. Have you prayed or meditated on working with this practitioner and gotten the go-ahead?

Once you have gone through the list and determined that this could be the right practitioner for you, set up an appointment and get started!

What It Actually Looks Like When Someone Restores Their Health

When you come in for the Quantum Response Technique initial consultation, your practitioner will gather a significant amount of information from you. During the assessment, she will find out more about your history and your goals. Because your body collects information and records everything that has ever happened to you, your entire history is important.

The practitioner will recommend assessments or tests based on your goals. Most people who come to our office get muscle testing for a baseline of information and an initial action plan.

The practitioner will then take the information she has collected from you and the goals you have indicated to create a program specifically for you. She will not jump into a complete recommendation in the first appointment but will take time after your appointment to review your information and consider your options.

You will get the recommendations in your report of findings appointment. We recommend that you bring a trusted friend or spouse to the report of findings since many people find it helpful to have a second pair of ears when making important health decisions.

Some of the options you will be given:

- **Quantum Response Testing** is muscle testing that allows the practitioner to ask your body the nuances of what it needs as it changes. This is best for people who are open-minded, committed to improving their health, and willing to make lifestyle changes. Your practitioner works closely with you and is best for people with significant health issues. The more significant your health issue, the more frequent the visits and the more intensive the program. You will always start with supplements to support your detoxification and digestion. Quantum Response Testing is the secret behind what brings people to level 4 health. (Wellness visits are available for those who want to check in with the feedback of muscle testing, but don't need the close support in QRT.)

- **The Nutrition Master Class** is a self-directed program that focuses on how to keep your diet and your environment as healthy as possible. It cuts through the fads and trends to the foundation of what food habits cause your body to be healthy. If you think your diet is healthy, but you aren't sure or are curious if what you do know will optimize your health, you can take a self-assessment at www. NutritionReadinessQuiz.com. In the Nutrition Master Class, you are guided toward doable changes, advised on how to handle common challenges, and set up for lifelong improvement. Since around 60 to 70 percent of your healing depends on what you put in your body, this is one of the most important programs we offer.

- **Emotional & Mental Balancing & Repatterning (EMBeR)** is an option anywhere along your recovery process. In the initial session, you identify stressors in your environment and make a plan for lessening or removing them. You are also given tools for removing the emotional blocks that are hindering you from making healthy choices. Subsequent visits with a practitioner help you dig deeper for the "big ones" that are hard to get to on your own.

- **Detoxification foot baths** gently support your body in removing toxins. Local patients often enjoy coming into the office. The footbaths can also be ordered for home use. Quality matters, so we only offer the best in our office.

- **Functional medicine tests** are familiar tests for most people since most of the tests are blood tests. Pathogens and gastrointestinal imbalances can be found in your stool sample. Hormone imbalances can be found in your saliva. There are many possibilities. Because the tests are not dictated by the confines of insurance policies, your practitioner has the freedom to listen to you and make the best recommendations for you. The information from these tests allows us to determine important supplementation that will support your body for improvement. Usually, you take the recommendations for three months to a year, and then retest to determine what your next nutritional supplementation recommendations will be.

Functional Medicine Testing vs. Muscle Testing

Functional medicine tests allow us to see the big picture. Muscle testing allows us to see the big picture from a different perspective and also allows us to see the nuances that your body needs as it changes. We can meet the changes of your body's needs every step of the way. Muscle testing is also excellent for an out-of-the-box healthy pregnancy because nothing changes as much or as quickly as the creation of a new human being.

The focus at the beginning of your Quantum Response Testing program is improved digestion and the removal of interferences. Continual detoxification may be necessary given the high level of pollution in our world. However, the number of supplements needed for detoxification usually decreases over time with improved lifestyle choices.

As your health and diet improve, supplements are added for organ support and overall health. Visits are weekly for the first few months to ensure that the changes your body is trying to make are supported with the appropriate nutrients.

Depending on the amount of damage in your body, you may need up to twenty or more different types of supplements at any one time. Some people with significant damage to their organs have been able to restore their health on as few as six supplements. They did this by taking charge of and significantly improving their diet, having a loving community that supported them in their dietary and environmental changes, and having a strong spiritual life.

People who have already begun implementing the recommended nutritional changes have quicker and more significant results. This is why many people choose to start with the Nutrition Master Class.

During the first week of Quantum Response Testing, you will start taking your supplements. You will also begin nutrition coaching if you haven't already.

During the second week, you start with your footbath series.

You will have weekly QRT visits for the first few months. Your supplements and their dosages will change most weeks. Your practitioner will give you tips on your diet. You are expected to make your best effort to implement changes and stay in communication with your practitioner.

At about four weeks in, you should start noticing changes.

You are feeling better. In week 5, you are tracking your food and noticing that your heart races about four days after you ate some blueberries. You have made the connection between fruit sugar and your symptoms. You will not be eating fruit again until the muscle testing indicates that the body is no longer this sensitive to it.

Over time, you continue identifying healthy foods, playing the "poison game" while grocery shopping, and are feeling like a new person.

Over the first few weeks, you start eating healthier foods while avoiding dairy and fruits. At month 4, you are able to reintroduce fruit—and it isn't messing you up like it used to!

You still hold off on the dairy, but know that you may be able to use it again.

You've started meditating and are facing the day calmer and happier. It helps that your stomach isn't bothering you.

The next step is to give your heart the nutrients it needs. You know that your body runs on food, so you use high-quality, food-based supplements. You are taking the supplements made from organ meats—if you need to heal your heart, you eat heart—or take the supplement if you don't want to eat a heart.

Your body starts to feel better and you have more energy. Your blood pressure starts to normalize and you are no longer borderline diabetic.

Your medical doctor reduces your blood pressure medications and tells you to "keep doing what you are doing."

You slowly get more toxins out of your environment. You start taking thyroid restoring supplements.

You realize that your diet is key to your health. You know that if you eat the things your body doesn't like, you notice your symptoms. Perhaps your blood pressure goes back up or your thyroid starts feeling funny.

You notice that any time you expose yourself to a toxin or something that bothers your body, your symptoms come back or you get new symptoms. You are getting reconnected with your innate wisdom.

As you move forward, you decide that you want these organs optimized. You continue to work on getting your mind in the right place, you exercise regularly, and you are kinder and kinder to yourself.

At the three-year mark, you are off your medications and are taking supplements to support your organs.

Since you live in the country, you know you need detoxification support during harvesting season. (If you're in the city, you need this for pollution.)

You have a filter for your water. You are clear about what you need to do to stay healthy. You have learned how to muscle test and can use that for yourself and your family for basic things like choosing the right thing for when your child gets sick, deciding what to have for dinner, or other choices that may affect your mental, emotional, or spiritual health.

You are very clear on what keeps you healthy and what makes you sick. You are out of the medical system. Sometimes you have setbacks due to the stresses of life, but you know what to do when that happens. Your health is maximized, and you know how to keep it that way. You are successfully fighting off the natural aging process.

You have clarity, certainty and peace about your health and the future of your health.

Resources

Resources mentioned in this book are available at www.vimandvigorbook.com/resources. You can download some of them directly at the following websites.

If you would like my recommended list of whole food supplements for general support as well as detoxification, go to www.WholeFoodSupplementList.com.

If you would like a list of how to tell if the nutrients in your vitamins and supplements are synthetic or natural, go to www.WhatsInMyPills.com.

If you want to check your knowledge on what is healthy eating, you can take the free Nutrition Readiness Quiz at www.NutritionReadinessQuiz.com.

If you want to find out more about the basics of muscle testing, you can get a free download at www.muscletestingbasics.com.

For a list of some of the more common chemicals and metals you will see in your life, you can get the list at www.ToxinsInMyLife.com. The detox footbath I recommend is also there.

Books

Available for download at www.DrBonnieJuul.com:

Visualization to Manifestation: Why most visualizations fail and how to make yours succeed

Intuition, Faith, and Freedom: The one at-home tool you need to avoid using medical intervention

End Notes

Chapter 3

Raj Kumar, Arushi Kumar, Jayesh Srdhara. Pineal Gland—A Spiritual Third Eye: An Odyssey of Antiquity to Modern Chronomedecine. *Indian Journal of Neurosurgery* 2018;7:1–4, Department of Neurosurgery, Sanjay Gandhi Postgraduate Institute of Medical Sciences, Lucknow, Uttar Pradesh, India.

E. Kalisinska, I. Bosiacka-Baranowska, N. Lanocha, and colleagues. Fluoride Concentrations in the Pineal Gland, Brain and Bone of Goosander (Mergus Merganser) and Its Prey in Odra River Estuary in Poland. *Environmental Geochemistry and Health* 2014;36(6), 1063–1077. https://doi.org/10.1007/s10653-014-9615-6

Chapter 4

The Water in You: Water and the Human Body, US Geological Survey (usgs.gov).

Chapter 5

Sally Fallon Morell discussed the importance of animal fats in her book, *Nourishing Fats: Why We Need Animal Fats for Health and Happiness.*

David U. Himmelstein, Robert M. Lawless, Deborah Thorne, Pamela Foohey, and Steffie Woolhandler. Medical Bankruptcy: Still Common Despite the Affordable Care Act. *American Journal of Public Health* 2019:109, 431–433, https://doi.org/10.2105/AJPH.2018.304901

Poverty Among the Population Aged 65 and Older (fas.org).

Weston A. Price, *Nutrition and Physical Degeneration.*

Paul Pitchford, *Healing with Whole Foods: Oriental Traditions and Modern Nutrition.*

Emilie Raffa, *Artisan Sourdough Made Simple: A Beginner's Guide to Delicious Handcrafted Bread with Minimal Kneading.*

Chapter 6

Environmental Working Group, www.EWG.org

Your Diet Soda Habit May Raise Stroke, Dementia Risk (aarp.org)

How high fructose intake may trigger fatty liver disease, National Institutes of Health (NIH)

Israa T. Ismail, Oliver Fiehn and colleagues. Sugar Alcohols Have a Key Role in Pathogenesis of Chronic Liver Disease and Hepatocellular Carcinoma in Whole Blood and Liver Tissues, *Cancer*, 2020 Feb 19; 12(2):484.

P. De Cock, Erythritol Functional Roles in Oral-Systemic Health, *Adv Dent Res*, 2018 (Feb;29(1):104-109.

Toxic Exposure: Chemicals are in our water, food, air and furniture, University of California

Chapter 7

The Water in You: Water and the Human Body, US Geological Survey (usgs.gov).

Chapter 8

Modern farming practices: www.californiaearthminerals.com/media/mineral-nutrient-depletion-in-us-farm-and-range-soils.pdf

Vaccinations and the MTHFR mutation: There has literally been only one study ever done on MTHFR and vaccination side effects. The medical community can, as they do in this article in *Genetic Lifehacks*, state that there is no research showing a link between MTHFR gene mutations and vaccines. Because there are literally no studies. (Well, there was one many years ago.) However, there are patterns that those of us observing from outside the system see. And there is a pattern of bad reactions and the MTHFR gene mutation. This is considered, unfortunately, anecdotal evidence and considered invalid. Hopefully, you recognize a significant disconnect with the reasoning. The gene mutation test is fairly simple for you to get from many alternative health providers.

About the Author

Bonnie Juul is a chiropractor with advanced training in advanced muscle testing techniques, nutrition, emotional healing, aging, and longevity. She earned her doctor of chiropractic degree from Parker University in Dallas, Texas.

She has practitioner training and experience in Nutrition Response Testing, Emotional Freedom Technique, The Journey, Reiki, NeuroEmotional Technique, PSYH-K, Wholistic Kinesiology, Body Energetic Technique, and Yoga for Chakra Opening.

Her educational background also includes a bachelor of science degree in health and wellness, a bachelor of science in anatomy.

Dr. Bonnie is the founder of Quantum Response Technique, Quantum Response Testing and EMBeR or Emotional & Mental Balancing & Repatterning.

Her vision is to shift the paradigm of health to one of longevity and vitality with a respect for and understanding of innate wisdom and personal choice.

Her practice is based in Carbondale, Illinois, and St. Louis, Missouri, and she can be contacted through her website at www.naturalhealthwins.com.

I've done what I'm supposed to. Why is something still wrong with me?

Are you looking for healthcare answers in a broken medical delivery system? Tired of the emotional roller coaster, doctors' visits, medications, and more medications? Are you seeking solutions to just not feeling well but never getting a straight answer and only minimal help from mainstream health providers? You've been called a hypochondriac or crazy or just unreasonable? You don't know what the truth is.

You believe your body was designed to be healthy. You're *supposed* to be healthy.

You're mad or frustrated and you want out. You've said, "I can't do this anymore!" And you've prayed for help.

At the end of the frustration lie answers and people who have forged and walked the path out and into a place where doctors' visits are focused on what you seek:

- Ever-increasing health, vitality, and longevity,

- Where the aging among us look younger than everyone else in their age group, and are more active, and

- Where children are climbing trees and playing with bugs and with each other rather than having emotional outbursts and temper tantrums in grocery stores.

Those on the outside of this world look at them and say these people are lucky.

No, they aren't. They have a plan. And a strategy. And the solution is in the pages of this book.

Dr. Bonnie Juul is a chiropractor with advanced training in advanced muscle testing techniques, nutrition, emotional healing, aging, and longevity.

Made in the USA
Middletown, DE
20 November 2022

15089836R00109